Beautiful Eyes

Beautiful Eyes

Consumer's Guide to Cosmetic Eyelid Surgery (Second Edition)

Joseph A. Mauriello, Jr, MD
Oculoplastic Surgeon

EYELIDMD.NET
Summit, New Jersey 07901
Sea Girt, New Jersey 08750

Writers Club Press
New York Lincoln Shanghai

Beautiful Eyes
Consumer's Guide to Cosmetic Eyelid Surgery
(Second Edition)

Writers Club Press
an imprint of iUniverse, Inc.

For information address:
iUniverse, Inc.
2021 Pine Lake Road, Suite 100
Lincoln, NE 68512
www.iuniverse.com

Please note that the information contained in this book is educational. It does intend to constitute a second opinion or to create a physician-patient relationship. Also, it is not intended to violate any pre-existing physician-patient relationship.

ISBN: 0-595-16846-9

Printed in the United States of America

This book is dedicated to my wife, Marilyn, and to all people whose "Beautiful Eyes" are only matched by the goodness of their hearts.

CONTENTS

PREFACE

Purpose of cosmetic eyelid surgery: What is the first thing you notice when you look at a person's face? Most people will answer, "the eyes." This book outlines the components of "beautiful eyes" but really concerns "beautiful eyelids" that frame the eyes. Beautiful eyes are appreciated with age as long as they are visible and not obscured by the sagging skin of the upper eyelids or asymmetric, baggy lower eyelids. Eyes brighten and are opened wider when drooping, excess skin is removed. Since 1983, Dr. Mauriello, a board certified ophthalmologist, has dedicated his career to oculoplastic surgery (eyelid, tear duct, socket, and orbital surgery). A member of the American society of Ophthalmic Plastic and Reconstructive Surgery, Dr. Mauriello has developed cosmetic eyelid techniques to enhance patient results.

Any distortion of the eyelids detracts from the observer's view of the eyes. Eyes brighten and appear more opened after cosmetic, restorative eyelid surgery. The techniques outlined in the book do not change the shape of the eyes. Dr. Mauriello's patients who undergo eyelid surgery are grateful for subtle changes that dramatically restore the upper face.

In this book, Dr. Mauriello provides his patients' critique of their results in order to satisfy himself that the surgical results are continuing to benefit his patients. Patients have told Dr. Mauriello that his techniques produce consistent, natural results. Patients do not complain of scarring or changing the shape of the eyelids after cosmetic eyelid surgery.

The term "cosmetic surgery" is defined in Stedman's Medical dictionary as a surgical operation that will improve the appearance of a person or prevent disfigurement. Dr. Mauriello believes that cosmetic eyelid surgery is restorative surgery that results in a refreshed appearance and does not create a plastic appearance. Rather in its purest form, it **restores** a youthful appearance.

Cosmetic upper lid surgery: The upper lid requires a defined, natural crease with a fold of skin that symmetrically overhangs that crease. Age-related loss of a well-defined upper eyelid crease occurs. The crease may be surgically reformed and sharpened to rejuvenate the eyelids without changing their natural appearance. Excess loose, aged skin that overhangs the upper eyelid crease is removed in a conservative fashion. Fat that bulges unevenly in the upper and lower lids may be surgically excised or flattened in order to create symmetry and achieve a refreshed look. After all, what physical structure such as a car or home does not need occasional maintenance and, eventually, structural support after 30 to 50 years? *Dr. Mauriello reviews photographs of patients taken when young in order to restore their eyelids.*

Cosmetic lower lid surgery: Dr. Mauriello has developed surgical techniques that remove excess skin and bags and also elevate the upper cheek fat pad. All the surgery is performed through a tiny skin incision in the corner of eye. An incision that goes across the entire lower eyelid is not required.

Botox and Restylane: Office Botox® treatments maintain results in the upper face while Restylane® improves the wrinkles in the lower face. No matter what effort is taken to minimize aging, all rejuvenation efforts are satisfying and can dramatically improve the individual's appearance.

SCOPE OF "BEAUTIFUL EYES"

This book is written for individuals who are considering cosmetic eyelid surgery and wish to be educated. Its main goal is to make information available to you. It is written so that you will be able to review the various sections of book at your leisure rather than in a relatively short surgical consultation or from a friend who may have undergone previous cosmetic surgery. Well-meaning friends may unfortunately provide misleading information. *"Beautiful Eyes" teaches you that your eyelids have a unique structure and any appropriate surgery must consider this uniqueness.* While no reading material replaces the intimacy and one-on-one benefits of a pre-surgical consultation, this text helps you determine whether you are a candidate for cosmetic surgery and provides you with pertinent questions to present to the surgeon at the of your consultation. A glossary in the Appendix at the end of the book refreshes the reader about meanings of medical terms that are defined throughout the book.

Definitions of blepharoplasty The term blepharoplasty (cosmetic eyelid surgery) is derived from "blepharo" which means eyelid and "plasty" which is defined in Stedman's medical dictionary as a surgical procedure for repair of a defect and restoration of a part. Ultimately, "plasty" denotes form and shape and, therefore, has functional implications. Blepharoplasty surgically restores form and function to the eyelids. The approach of plastic surgery is increasingly restorative rather than transforming. Most patients wish revitalization without looking different especially in the eyelid area. While patients may wish to change the shape of their nose through surgery, Dr. Mauriello has found that patients do not wish to change the shape of their eyes. A possible exception is the rare Asian patient who may desire a change to a westernized or caucasian upper eyelid crease.

Types of doctors who perform such surgery Various types of surgeons perform cosmetic eyelid surgery or "cosmetic blepharoplasty." This book is written by an oculoplastic surgeon, a board certified ophthalmologist specializing in eyelid surgery. *Because of their in-depth knowledge of the eye and the eyelids, ophthalmic plastic and reconstructive (oculoplastic) surgeons such as Dr. Mauriello offer their patients the highest level of specialization that are blended with technical skills and an artistic sense to create a functioning and well proportioned anatomic unit.*

Outline of book: This book outlines the necessary steps in surgical care necessary to achieve beautiful eyes. The various chapters help you:

- determine whether you are a candidate for cosmetic eyelid surgery
- select a surgeon
- understand the various cosmetic eyelid and skin rejuvenating procedures
- follow the entire surgical process, step by step, from the pre-surgical consultation to the post-operative care including maintenance of long-term results

The book categorizes structural eyelid changes that occur with age:
30 to 55 years of age: minimal excess skin is present in the upper eyelid along with some bulging of fat in the lower eyelid.
50 to 70 years of age: the gravitational effects of aging become more pronounced with drooping of the outer aspect of the eyebrows

often becomes evident. The upper cheek fat pad descends and the bone under the eye is exposed and circles appear under the eyes

70 years of age or older: all changes that occur in the earlier stages are present. In addition, there may be drooping of the upper eyelid margin (blepharoptosis) due to thinning of the tendon (aponeurosis) of the levator muscle and exaggerated brow droop (brow ptosis). The outer corners of the eyes become blunted. There is progressive loss of the elasticity of the skin and laxity of the supporting eyelid ligaments. There is also thinning or atrophy of the muscle. Thinning (atrophy) of the fat and loss of volume in the facial tissues produce the skeletonized look of aging. Descent of the cheek becomes increasingly evident.

Aging is to a large degree genetically determined, but other environmental factors such as sun exposure, cigarette smoking, and underlying disease also have considerable influence. Questions are posed in each chapter and answered in the text. In this manner, the necessary elements to achieve beautiful eyes are provided to the reader. *This book provides information that is not available anywhere else.*

After surgery, Dr. Mauriello's patients are asked to respond to a questionnaire of frequently asked questions. The patients' responses are recorded in the book in the form of testimonials. Dr. Mauriello has found that many patients are enthusiastic about the results of his surgery but virtually all patients are extremely satisfied. Furthermore, the eyelids are an isolated unit of the face with unique features. For example, the eyelid skin is the only area in the body where muscle underlines the skin rather than fat. The eyelid area and upper cheek may be surgically rejuvenated using Dr. Mauriello's techniques and the results are long lasting. Facelifts involve mobilizing larger anatomic units of the face and generally do not last as long as the eyelid surgery.

Autobiographical note

Joseph A. Mauriello, Jr, MD is one of a handful of board certified ophthalmologists in Northern New Jersey who specializes in ophthalmic plastic and reconstructive (oculoplastic) surgery that involves eyelid as well as tear duct, socket, or orbital surgery. Dr. Mauriello, Director of Oculoplastic Surgery at UMD-NJ Medical School at Newark from 1983 to 1998, was one of the first ophthalmologists to dedicate his entire medical practice to Oculoplastic surgery in New Jersey. He is, therefore, in a unique position to educate the patient. Since 1998, he has dedicated his practice almost exclusively to cosmetic eyelid surgery. He maintains office in Summit and in Sea Girt at the Jersey Shore. *Cosmetic eyelid surgery is the only cosmetic surgery Dr. Mauriello performs.*

About Dr. Mauriello's Training

*   Medical school training at UMD—New Jersey Medical School, Newark, NJ 1972–76

*   Medical internship at Overlook Hospital, Summit, NJ (affiliate of Columbia Presbyterian College of Physicans and Surgeons in 1977

*   Ophthalmology residency at New York University Medical Center, 1977–80

Dr. Mauriello received a two-year training grant from the National Eye Institute for a Fellowship in ophthalmic pathology at the Armed Forces Institute of Pathology (AFIP) from 1980–82. The AFIP has 39 branches and serves as a consultative pathology center for the armed forces but also for civilian pathologists. The Ophthalmic Pathology branch at the AFIP is world renown and has a long tradition of excellence in teaching and in diagnosing tissue specimens from the eye, eyelids, orbit, and lacrimal system.

Dr. Mauriello trained in ophthalmic plastic and reconstructive surgery (oculoplastic surgery) at Wills Eye Hospital in Philadelphia in 1982–83. This training was supported by a one-year grant awarded by the Heed Ophthalmic Foundation in Chicago. This foundation provides stipends for promising young investigators who pursue advanced subspecialty training in ophthalmology.

While there are no subspecialty boards in ophthalmology or oculoplastic surgery, the American Society of Ophthalmic Plastic and Reconstructive Surgery (ASOPRS.org) elects candidates as Fellows who complete four years of medical school, a one-year internship, a three year residency in ophthalmology, and finally a two year fellowship approved by the ASOPRS' organization. In addition, after completing an approved fellowship in ophthalmic plastic and reconstructive surgery, the candidate must write a thesis that is approved by the Thesis Committee and then pass both written and oral examinations in order to gain membership as fellows in the society.

About Dr. Mauriello's Experience: Dr. Mauriello was also honored to be selected as one of the *BEST DOCTORS OF AMERICA (1998–2004)* according to the input of 35,000 physicians. *The Best Doctors in American (bestdoctors.com) is based on two year surveys both locally and nationally performed by Woodward/White.* He received the American Academy of Ophthalmology *Honor Award* in 1991 for his scientific contributions to the Academy. He has published with over 70 original articles in peer-reviewed journals and, in addition, published 30 chapters in scientific books. Dr. Mauriello was also elected to the international Orbital Society, an esteemed group of 25 members in 1994. He is a reviewer for many of the major ophthalmologic journals. Dr. Mauriello was asked to serve on the Medical Advisory Board of the American Society of Ocularists in 2000–2003. He is honored to have served as a member of the Editorial Board of the Ophthalmic Plastic and Reconstructive Surgery (OPRS) Journal since 2003.

Dr. Mauriello is a fellow member of **the American Society of Opthalmic Plastic and Reconstructive Surgery** and **the American Academy of Cosmetic Surgery.** He has presented over 100 papers at national meetings and has been selected for panels on national symposia throughout his career in order to help inform surgical colleagues. Dr. Mauriello's first textbook, *Management of Orbital and Ocular Adnexal Tumors and Inflammations*, was co-authored by Dr. Joseph C. Flanagan, Director of Oculoplastic Surgery, at Wills Eye Hospital, Philadelphia, Pa. He completed editing his second major medical textbook concerning eyelid and lacrimal surgery. The book has a separate section dedicated to cosmetic forehead, eyelid, and midfacial cosmetic surgery as well as laser resurfacing. Each chapter contains expert commentary by over 175 national and international specialists in oculoplastic surgery, dermatology, plastic surgery, and otolaryngology. Butterworth Heineman, the international medical publisher in Boston, published this 595-page text in the summer of 2000. His third book, *Techniques of Cosmetic Eyelid Surgery: A case study approach* Lippincott, Williams & Wilkins, Philadelphia, PA, was published in 2004. The present text, *Beautiful Eyes (2nd Edition),* is an attempt to inform the public about changes in cosmetic eyelid surgery.

Dr. Mauriello has been a member of Education Committee of the American Society of Ophthalmic Plastic and Reconstructive Surgery (ASOPRS) for over a decade. He has composed questions for the written examination for the society and acted as an oral examiner for prospective candidates prior to their acceptance into the Society. He has also served as one of four members on the Thesis Committee who evaluates candidates' theses for membership in ASOPRS and was chairman in 2002. Since 2003, he is honored to have served as Chair of the Continuing Medical Education Committee.

Joseph A. Mauriello, Jr, MD
Ophthalmic Plastic and Reconstructive Surgery
Fellow, American Society of Ophthalmic Plastic and Reconstructive Surgery
Fellow, American Academy of Ophthalmology (board certified Ophthalmologist)
Fellow, American Academy of Cosmetic Surgery

Cosmetic Eyelid and Facial Rejuvenation Center
33 Overlook Road   2130 Route 35
Suite 104   Suite 115-A
Summit, NJ 07901   Sea Girt, NJ 08750
908-608-1200   732-449-3299
URL: EYELIDMD.NET

Section 1

INTRODUCTION

CHAPTER 1

Am I a candidate for eyelid rejuvenation?
Eyelid Anatomy
The Stages of Eyelid Aging

This section answers all your questions about whether you are a candidate for cosmetic eyelid surgery and also considers the basic *Anatomy of the Eyelid* and the *Stages of Eyelid Aging*.

Importance of Cosmetic Surgery in the United States, 2004
According to *Cosmetic Surgery Times (April, 2004)*, total surgical and non-surgical procedures included over 8 million in 2003 as compared to slightly more than 2 million in 1997 (data obtained from the American Society of Aesthetic Plastic Surgeons).
Liposuction was the most popular surgical cosmetic procedure, with more than 380,000 surgeries in 2003. More than 60,000 such procedures were requested by men who, like woman, wish to maintain a youthful appearance for social and career-based reasons.
Five Most Popular Surgical Cosmetic Procedures in 2003
Liposuction   384,626
Breast augmentation   280,401

Eyelid surgery	267,627
Rhinoplasty	172,420
Female breast reduction	147,173

Botox continues to be the most popular cosmetic office procedure. Restylane is a natural filler of facial creases particularly in the lower portion of the face and it has virtually supplanted collagen since no skin testing is necessary and it lasts longer than collagen (6 months or longer).

Top Nonsurgical Cosmetic Procedures

Botox Injection	2,272,080
Laser Hair Removal	923,200
Microdermabrasion	858,312
Chemical Peel	722,248
Collagen Injection	620,476

The total number of surgical and nonsurgical Procedures for each year are as follows:

1997	2.1 Million
2002	6.9 Million
2003	8.3 Million

The above statistics do not include those of other societies including the American Society of Ophthalmic Plastic and Reconstructive Surgery (ASOPRS.org, board certified ophthalmologists), the American Academy of Cosmetic Surgery (board certified cosmetic surgeries of multiple disciplines) including ophthalmologists, board certified oto-laryngologists (American Academy of Facial Plastic Surgery), and board certified dermatologists (American Academy of Dermatology).

Eyelid surgery results in great improvement that is long-lasting. According to a McCall's magazine article, "10 years after plastic surgery...What are the long-term results? Real women tell the truth about life after the knife" (November, 2000). A patient who underwent cosmetic eyelid surgery stated that: "my eyes still look great ten years later." Cosmetic eyelid surgery, in Dr. Mauriello's experience, restores the entire face. His patients attest to the fact that tired eyes are improved by his techniques.

Studies show that cosmetic surgery has a dramatic effect on the individual's psyche and lifestyle (Sarwer DB. Health Professionals need a new perspective on cosmetic surgery *Aesthetic Surg* J. 0:223-224, 2000). Fifty-six per cent of American women are not satisfied with their overall appearance. The importance of physical appearance on interpersonal and social interactions is crucial and cosmetic surgery helps alleviate symptoms of depression and quality of life and body image problems (Garner DM. The 1997 body image survey results. *Psychology Today* 1997: 31: 30-87). The results can be dramatic and exhilarating for the both patient the surgeon.

After performing thousands of eyelid surgery, Dr. Joseph Mauriello has found that many patients are enthusiastic about the results. Virtually all patients are extremely satisfied. *Furthermore, since the eyelids are an isolated unit of the face, the area may be surgically restored and the results last 10 years or longer. Facelifts involve mobilizing larger anatomic units of the face and generally do not last as long as the eyelid surgery.*

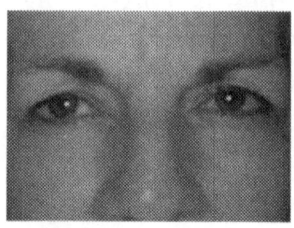 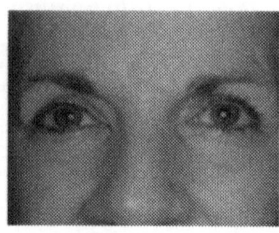 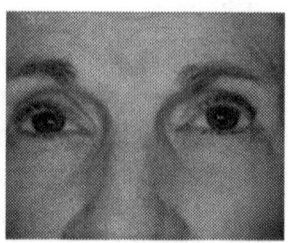

Figure 1
58 year-old woman
prior to upper lid
blepharoplasty

Figure 2
Improvement 3
months after surgery

Figure 3
12 years after surgery

Why consider cosmetic eyelid surgery?

Beautiful Eyes can be yours. Cosmetic eyelid surgery removes excess skin in the upper and lower eyelids as well as unsightly bulges of fat that protrude through the skin. The effect after surgery is create symmetry and "clean" lines that allow people to look directly into your most natural asset, your "Beautiful Eyes." Eyelid surgery improves your entire appearance by creating improved symmetry of the eyelids. Patients comment that the surgery appears to open the eyes. After surgery, the focus of attention becomes your expressive eyes. Eyelid surgery rejuvenates and actually restores the entire face without the downtime associated with more extensive procedures such as the face lift. The eyelid surgery may be enhanced by appropriate skin care and other office facial rejuvenation procedures (Botox®, wrinkle-fillers such as Restylane®).

> *Dr. Mauriello has developed special techniques that actually elevate the cheek at the same time excess lower lid skin and lower lid bags are removed.*

By answering the following questions, you may determine whether you are a candidate for upper or lower cosmetic eyelid surgery.

1. *Do you look tired in the morning even after you take a nap?*
    There is more swelling in the eyelids especially after lying flat in bed all night. This dependent fluid dissipates as the day wears on. Due to aging, the eyelid skin sags and bulges beyond a certain critical point such that no amount of sleep will relieve the tired appearance.

2. *Are you in a competitive working environment where age, looks, and communication count?*
    A youthful, less tired appearance is extremely important in the working environment today. Whether you work or stay at home with your family, you will look, feel, and possibly perform better after cosmetic eyelid surgery. Attractive people receive preferential treatment in our society. Less attractive people do not command as much attention. Baggy and sagging eyelids and depressed cheeks take focus away from your eyes.

3. *Do either of my parents or siblings have drooping eyelids and do I wish to have similar appearing lids at their particular age?*
    By simply viewing other members of the family, particularly one of your parents whose eyelids resemble yours, you can predict with a fair degree of certainty how you will look with age.

4. *Do you feel extra weight on your eyelids and when you manually lift the eyelid skin with your fingers is the "heaviness" temporarily relieved?*
    Excess skin above the eyelid crease that overhangs the eyelashes create heaviness similar to "fish weights" on the upper eyelids. The skin folds rub against themselves and may cause redness and itching. Most

commonly, a combination of such factors interferes with reading, watching television, and driving a car. Does manually lifting the upper eyelids with your fingers relieve the symptoms? When the eyelid tissues contribute significantly to such functional complaints, medical insurance may reimburse patients for upper lid surgery.

5. *Are there horizontal lines in the forehead?*
A special muscle in the forehead (the frontalis muscle) elevates the eyebrows and heavy upper eyelids so that vision is improved. You may notice horizontal forehead lines and that your eyebrows are constantly elevated in order to compensate for the weighted-down heavy upper eyelid tissues. Ultimately, the eyelids become increasingly heavy over time and you may become fatigued after reading for only a brief period of time.

6. *Do you get tired after reading for as short as only a few minutes or as long as an hour due to heaviness of the your upper eyelids? Do you sometimes get headaches by the end of the day especially when reading?*
A frontal (forehead) headache may occur by the end of the day by constantly raising the eyebrows in order to elevate the heavy upper eyelids. Similarly, one's leg would be sore if one stood on one leg all day. Headaches due to eye strain tend to occur at the end of the day or after a period of time due to eyestrain.

7. *Do you have problems seeing cars when driving especially out of the corner of one or both or your eyes?*
Peripheral vision may be blocked by excess eyelid skin which directly obscures part of the field of vision. Simply, lifting the uppers eyelid(s) with your fingers will simulates the effects of upper eyelid surgery. You may experience difficulty passing cars when driving due to decreased peripheral vision.

8. **Do I have bags below the eyes?**
   Baggy lower eyelids are especially bothersome to both women and men. These unsightly bulges are unacceptable and detract from your beautiful eyes. The lower eyelids and upper cheeks may be improved by Dr. Mauriello's techniques that are part of his routine cosmetic or restorative lower eyelid surgery.

9. **Do your eyes appear smaller?**
   The space between the upper and lower eyelid margins, known as the palpebral fissure, is the space occupied by the eye. This space narrows vertically with age. It also narrows horizontally due to loosening of the ligaments especially at the outer corners of the eyes. These distances may be increased with surgery.

10. **Do coworkers ask if you are tired when you are not?**
    If your response is positive to any of the above questions, you may benefit from eyelid surgery and may benefit from reading further.

EYELID ANATOMY

The eyelid skin is among the thinnest of the body. Just beneath the eyelid skin lies the orbicularis oculi muscle. *In other areas of the face and the body, there is intervening fat between the skin and the underlying muscle.* Due to the specialized function of the eyelids and their unique relationship to the eye, no intervening fat is present between the eyelid skin and the underlying musle. Furthermore, the tendons that support each eyelid are appropriately tightened and strengthened by your surgeon to enhance the effect of cosmetic eyelid surgery.

Cosmetic eyelid surgery correlate: Since the eyelids tissues contain muscle beneath their surface, any rearrangement of the tissue during cosmetic eyelid surgery tends to be *long-lasting*. The eyes and the surrounding lids are a separate compartment with unique anatomic features. Cosmetic eyelid surgery serves to tighten the muscle and skin together as one anatomic unit. This distance is quite short. The bulging fat beneath the eyelid muscle is treated separately from the skin muscle layers of the eyelids. In contrast, a face lift re-drapes heavy facial skin and underlying fasica and fat from distant incision sites behind and in front of the ear.

The orbicularis muscle of the eyelids wraps around the upper and lower eyelids in a circular fashion and acts like a sphincter to contract or close the eyelids. It has attachments known as raphes at the two corners of each eye. The inner corner of the eye is known as the medial canthus and the outer corner of the eye, the lateral canthus. These raphes or attachments act as fulcrums upon which the muscle contracts as a band of tissue to close the upper eyelid and lower eyelids. The tendons of the upper sand lower eyelid in the outer corner of the eye (the upper arms or crura of the lateral canthal tendon) attenuate or thin out with age and the eyelid structures become weakened. The weakening occurs to some extent due to sagging of the muscle and its attachments.

Blinking spreads the complex tear film across the surface of the eye and keeps the mucous membranes of the eye moist. In addition, the blink reflex as well as the bone that surrounds the eye serves to protect each eye from external injury. This bone encasement around each eye is known as the *orbit*.

Fat is present under the eyelid skin and orbicularis layers and the underlying levator muscle aponeurosis or fibrous tendon. The levator muscle elevates the upper eyelid (see below) while the orbicularis oculi muscle closes the eyelids.

Specialized eyelid anatomy near the eyelid margin
The layers of the eyelid near the eyelid margin of the upper and lower eyelids:

- eyelid skin

- orbicularis oculi muscle (closes the eye)

- tarsus or fibrous plate (provides support and structure to the eyelid near the eyelid margin. It contains meibomian oil glands that supply the tear film on the eye surface and help retard evaporation of the tears)

- conjunctiva (mucosal lining that rests against the eye).

The eyelid margin is a specialized structure where the protective skin layer on the outside of the eyelid meets the smooth mucosal lining of the eye, the conjunctiva. The eyelid margin is similar to a window sill in that it frames the eye.

The eyelashes normally arise from the front part of the eyelid at the eyelid margin. The blink reflex allows the lashes to keep foreign matter from entering the eye. The meibomian glands are located on the back portion of the eyelid margin immediately adjacent to the eye. The tiny almost microscopic openings of these meibomian glands are the final conduit for fatty sebaceous material, an essential component of the tear film which bathes the surface of the eye. This oily outer layer of the tear film arises from the fibrous tarsal plate of the eyelid. The tarsus serves as a support for the platform in the upper eyelid upon which woman place makeup.

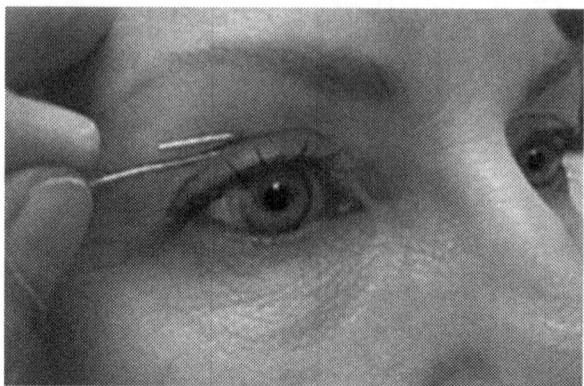

Figure 4—Crease is hiddened by fold of skin that is gently elevated by paper clip.

The individual photographed above is a candidate for cosmetic eyelid surgery. Note that the upper eyelid crease is not well dcfined. Excess skin, known as an *eyelid fold*, overhangs the *eyelid crease* that is gently exposed by bent paper clip in the photograph. The somewhat deep set eyes would only be accentuated by elevating the eyebrow. Careful and minimal excision of skin above the crease and surgical reformation of the eyelid crease is necessary to restore symmetric eyelids. This maneuver simulates the effect of the upper lid cosmetic surgery known as *upper blepharoplasty.*

The *lateral canthus* (outer corner of the eye) is normally 1–2 mm above the *medial canthus* (inner corner of the eye). Therefore, the outer corners of each eye are slightly higher than the inner corners. As stated above, the tarsus present in the upper and lower eyelids is the fibrous plate that supports the eyelids. The tarsus extends in the upper lid from the eyelid margin to the upper eyelid for 10 mm. In the lower lid, the tarsus has a vertical height 5 mm. The meibomian glands of the eyelid are the only sebaceous glands in the body that are not normally associated with hair follicles except under abnormal conditions. The meibomian glands retain this ability to produce abnormal lashes that arise from the back surface of the eyelids in a condition known as distichiasis. The most common cause of distichiasis is blepharitis, or inflammation of the eyelid margin that occurs commonly with age.

Upper eyelid above the tarsus

Movement of the upper lid is accomplished mainly by the levator muscle which extends from the back of the orbit about 18 mm (3/5 of an inch) behind the back of the eye and inserts on the upper tarsal border and also to the undersurface of the eyelid skin to create an upper eyelid crease. The upper eyelid crease is higher in females than males but is unique to each individual. The fold of skin above the crease may become exaggerated with age and is termed dermatochalasis (redundant skin).

Note that the fold of skin over eyelid crease is part of the male anatomy as well. Just in front of the levator muscle (and its tendon) is preaponeurotic fat. Orbital fat surrounds all orbital structures and is held in place by a thin fibrous investing structure known as the *orbital septum*. The orbital septum is in front of the preaponeurotic fat. When the orbital septum thins, the pre-aponeurotic and sometimes the deep orbital fat comes forward or prolapse especially in the nasal corner of the upper eyelid to create large bulges. The fat obliterates the eyelid crease in the upper eyelid. This fat is removed or repositioned and the upper lid crease reformed in cosmetic blepharoplasty.

Muscles that move the eyelids either directly or indirectly are striated muscles over which each individual has voluntary control. These muscles include the *levator muscle* that 5 mm opens the eye by elevating the upper eyelid. The orbicularis oculi muscle closes the eye, and extraocular muscles move the eyeball. In addition, the muscles of the eyebrow help close the eyes while the forehead musculature (*the frontalis muscle*) helps elevate the upper eyelid. Again, the frontalis muscle creates *horizontal lines* or furrows due to contraction of this vertically oriented muscle. There is also some elevation of the eyelid normally when this muscle contracts.

In addition to the levator muscle with its tendon or aponeurosis, the superior tarsal muscle, Muller's muscle, lies just beneath the conjunctiva also elevates the eyelid but only by 2mm. This involuntary muscle inserts at the upper tarsal border. It extends 10 mm (approximately 2/5 of an inch) vertically towards the rim of bone above the eye, known as the superior orbital rim. *Muller's muscle*, unlike the levator muscle, is not a voluntary (skeletal or striated muscle). Muller's muscle is a smooth (involuntary) muscle of the upper eyelid. Both the levator muscle and superior tarsal or Muller's muscle are known as upper eyelid retractors. Their antagonist muscles are the eyelid protractors that include the orbicularis muscle and the forehead muscles that depress the eyebrow. Such forehead muscles include the corrugator muscle that creates vertical frown lines and the procerus muscle or "muscle of menace" that pulls the eyebrow down towards to the base of the nose where it inserts. These vertical lines are best treated with Botox to weaken the muscle and Restylane® to fill any deep wrinkles.

Like the levator muscle, extraocular muscles arise from the back of the orbit (the orbital apex) and insert in the sclera of the eyeball to control the movement of the eye. The sclera is the white fibrous coat that protects and surrounds the delicate structures of the eye including the retina. The retina is a neural or brain-like tissue that sends visual data to the brain through the optic nerve.

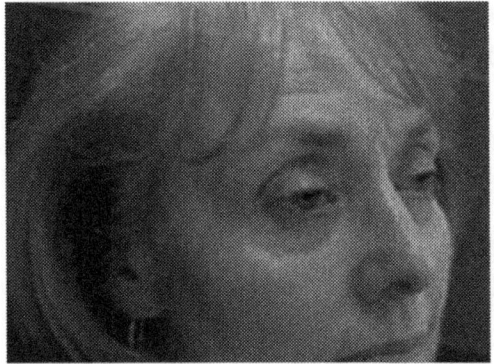

Figure 5

The patient photographed above has true upper lid ptosis such that the upper eyelid margin partially blocks the pupil. The horizontal lines in the forehead indicate that she uses the frontalis muscle in the forehead to elevate the eyelids and help compensate for the upper lid ptosis. She subsequently underwent repair of the droopy upper eyelids in order to improve visual function. After reading for short periods of time, she became fatigued and developed brow strain. The levator muscle tendon was tightened through an eyelid incision.

> *Editor's note: Lines in the forehead are often corrected by upper eyelid surgery. At times, Botox by relaxing the muscle improves such lines in patients who do not exhibit upper lid ptosis or excess heavy upper lid skin.*

Lower eyelid below the tarsal plate
The lower eyelid anatomy is similar to that of the upper eyelid.
The inferior rectus muscle is an extraocular muscle that attaches to the eye onto the white sclera at its lower surface. It pulls the eye downward. It inserts on the lower eyelid and has a so-called capsulopalpebral head, a tendon-like structure, which attaches the lower eyelid to the

inferior rectus muscle. The *capsulopalpebral head of the inferior rectus* (also known as the capsulopalpebral fascia) pulls or retracts the lower eyelid downward when the inferior rectus moves the eye downward. In this way, the eyeball and eyelid act in concert. The capsulopalpebral fascia is termed a lower eyelid retractor.

Like the superior tarsal muscle or Muller's muscle, the inferior tarsal muscle, a smooth involuntary muscle, lies just underneath the conjunctiva and on top of the capsulopalpebral fascia. It extends for 10 mm or approximately 2/5 of an inch. The inferiorly tarsal muscle inserts on the lower border of the tarsus (the platform or fibrous structure which provides support to the eyelid across the lower eyelid). The capsulopalpebral head of the inferior rectus muscle along with the inferior tarsal muscle pulls the eyelid downward. These the two structures, the capulsulopalpebral fascia and inferior tarsal muscle, constitute the two lower eyelid retractors and help pull the lower eyelid downward.

> *Editor's Note: Basically, the lower eyelid is attached to the eyeball and moves when the individual gazes downward.*

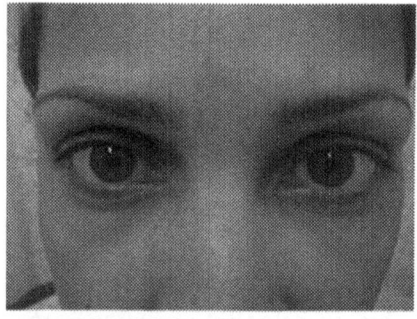

Figure 6
BEFORE

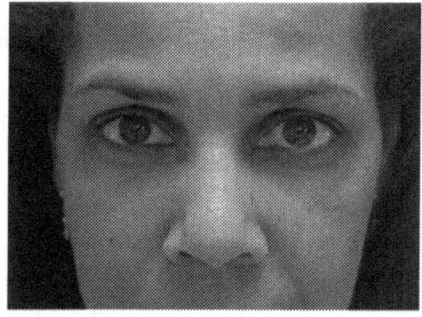

Figure 7
AFTER LOWER
BLEPHAROPLASTY

This patient (above right) complained that the eyeballs were getting larger, the lower lids were pulled down, and the upper cheeks were sagging with age. Note improvement after 3-step technique for lower blepharoplasty.

The orbit and its contents
The orbit has a volume of 30 cc, that of a shot glass. The orbit is demarcated by bone which has a fibrous inner coat known as the periorbita. The eye, itself, has a volume of approximately 7.5 cc and the remaining tissues in the orbit include:

*   the orbital fat that surrounds the muscles that move the eyeball

*   the muscle that move the eyes (extraocular muscles)

*   the myriad orbital nerves

*   the blood vessels that supply nutrients to these structures

The orbit is a highly complex but compact bony compartment that also protects the eyeball from outside external physical injury.

While extraocular muscles move the eyeball, the internal muscles of the eye include the iris constrictor and dilator and these muscles determine the size of the pupil, the open space within the iris. The ciliary muscle within the eye is responsible for accommodation or focusing at near.

Palpebral fissure: The palpebral fissure is the eyelid opening through which the cornea, the watchglass of the eye, focuses light on the retina. The retina lines the back internal surface of the eye.

Tarsus: The tarsus serves as a support for the platform in the upper eyelid upon which women place makeup.

Pupil and iris: The pupil is the dark or black hole in the center of the colored part of the eye, the iris. The pupil by changing its size allows light to focus on the retina. Again, the retina is the nerve tissue that analyzes light and transmits images to the brain so that the individual is able to see. If the pupil is covered by upper eyelid margin in severe ptosis, then vision is affected.

Conjunctiva: The conjunctiva, a thin clear layer of mucous membrane, lines the eyelid and eyeball's surface. It "conjoins" the eyelid to the eyeball as shown in the photograph below. The layer covers the back surface of the eyelid and lines the white supporting structure of the eyeball known as the sclera. In the photograph, the space between the inner surface of the eyelid and eyeball is known as the cul de sac. It is best seen when the lower eyelid is pulled down away from the eye.

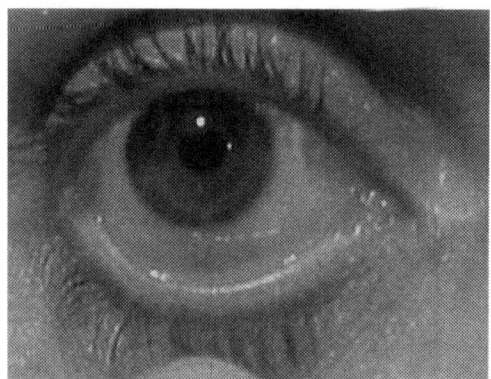

Figure 8
The *eyelid margin* with lashes emanating from its front portion is evident.

Lacrimal Drainage Apparatus: Each of the four eyelids have small openings called puncta. These openings lead to the tiny drains in the eyelid, the canaliculi, through which tears drain into the tear ducts. All these structures are in the inner most aspect of the eyelids on the side of the nose just nasal to where the eyelashes end. The canaliculi course on the upper and lower eyelid (medially by the nose) and drain in the lacrimal sac which is just below the medial canthus (nasal corner of the eye). The lacrimal sac drains through a bone structure known as the lacrimal canal via a mucosal lined membrane known as the naso-lacrimal duct on the side of the nose. Excess skin of the lower eyelid may stretch the lower eyelid and cause it to turn away from the front surface of the eyeball in an abnormal lid position known as **ectropion**. Tearing may result. Ectropion repair may be necessary at the time of the cosmetic blepharoplasty to restore normal tear drainage.

The Eyebrow: The eyebrow should begin on a line drawn parallel to the side of the nose to the protruding (frontal) bone above the eye. The eyebrow should end at line drawn from the outside of the nose by the nostril to the outer corner of the eye to intersect at the temple. The arch of the brow varies in each individual but, in general, starts at the outer edge of the iris, not at the pupil. The first 3/4 of the brow generally arches upward while the last quarter points downward. These anatomic considerations are important in any surgical approach to the eyebrow. They also apply to simple plucking the brow hairs to change the brow contour. The brows effectively frame the entire face and open the eyes. The highest point of the eyebrow is normally at the outer edge of the iris rather than at the center of the pupil. The ideal eyebrow starts from a point on a line drawn parallel to the side of the nose to the frontal bone above the eye.

> *Editorial note: The eyebrow position may be changed with Botox® or simply by careful brow plucking or tweezing of its hairs. Brow surgery is rarely recommended by Dr. Mauriello.*

STRUCTURAL EYELID CHANGES THAT ARE AGE RELATED

The structural eyelid changes are gravitational in nature and may be staged and categorized by age as shown below. Surgery is restorative rather than cosmetic.

FIRST STAGE—30 to 55 YEARS OF AGE

In the first stage, from 30 to 55 years of age, mild to moderate amounts of excess inelastic skin begins to hide the upper eyelid crease. Fat may bulge through the skin.

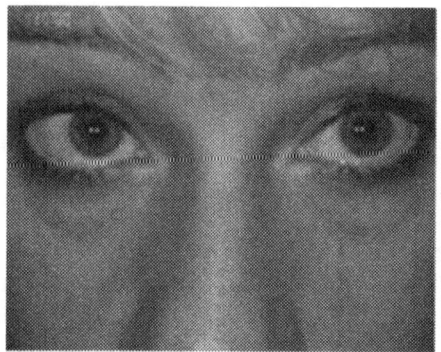
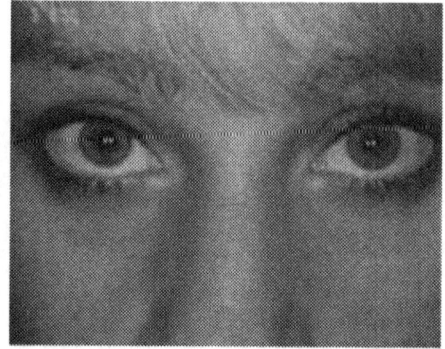

Figure 9
BEFORE

Figure 10
AFTER LOWER LID SURGERY

29 year-old with mild bulges of fat protruding through the lower eyelids more on the left than the patient's right side. Improvement of lower eyelid bulges after transconjunctival lower eyelid blepharoplasty. **No skin incisions or laser skin resurfacing were performed.** No upper eyelid surgery was necessary.

SECOND STAGE—AGES 50-70

The second stage consists of patients in their mid-fifties to early seventies. The above gravitational effects become more pronounced. The following patient has noted increased sagging of the skin and loss of skin turgor.

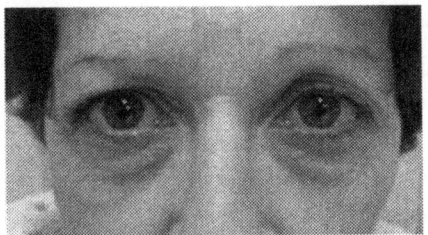 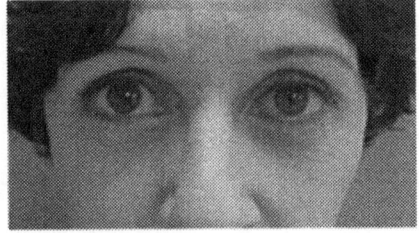

Figure 11   **Figure 12**
BEFORE   **AFTER 4 LID BLEPHAROPLASTY**

Patient has experienced greater symmetry of eyelids that frame and actually open the eyes. There is also cheek elevation.

> *Editor's Note: All eyelid surgery whether directed toward improved function or cosmesis only, when properly performed, yields improved cosmesis that open the eyes and focuses attentions on the eyes.*

> *Editorial note: Dr. Mauriello has special techniques to raise the upper cheek through a small incision in the outer corner of the eye. Scarring is rarely if ever a long-term problem after eyelid surgery because the eyelid skin is among the thinnest in the body and does not form thick scars or keloids.*

THIRD STAGE—OVER 70 YEARS OF AGE

In the third stage, over age 70, all of the above changes occur and in many patients there is actual of drooping upper eyelid margin (blepharoptosis) due to thinning of the tendon (aponeurosis) of the levator muscle and exaggerated brow droop (brow ptosis). The outer corners of the eyes becomes blunted. The progressive loss of the elasticity of the skin and in the supporting ligaments around the eye adds to the drooping eyelid skin. Fat atrophy in the face produces a skeletonized or emaciated appearance that accompanies old age. Finally, the fluid in the dermis of the eye, known as hyaluronic acid, decreases with age. This fluid creates the plump cheeks seen in babies. Restylane® is a synthetic form of hyaluronic acid that binds water in the tissues and plumps or refills wrinkles that occur with age.

Editor's note: Restylane® injections may be performed in office and produce remarkable results in the lower face. The results are prolonged by minute dosages of Botox®.

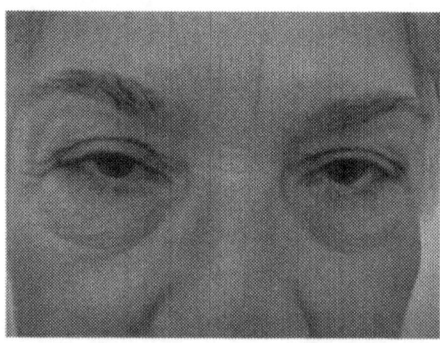

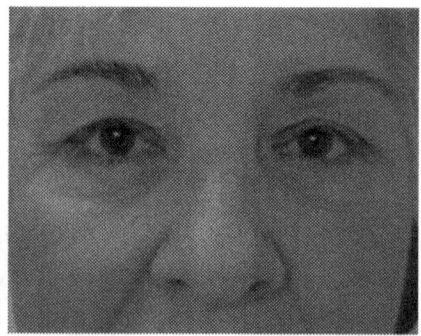

Figure 12
BEFORE SURGERY

Figure 13
AFTER UPPER LID PTOSIS
REPAIR AND 4-LID COSMETIC
BLEPHAROPLASTY

Patient in photograph (above left, BEFORE SURGERY) with severe right upper lid droop or ptosis since eyelid margin covers upper 1/3 of pupil. There is a moderate to severe blepharoptosis of the left upper eyelid since only the upper aspect of the pupil is covered. Excess skin covers the left upper eyelid crease. This excess skin needs to be excised because as the upper eyelids are elevated, there will be more skin overlying the eyelid margins due to an accordion-like effect. Since the upper lid skin extends beyond the outer corner of each eye, the upper eyelid skin incision will be made beyond the corner of the eye. This patient had evidence of levator dehiscence. There is marked fat that bulges in the lower eyelid. Surgical alternatives for patients with aging eyelids are discussed detail in: Chapter 3: What types of Cosmetic Eyelid and Upper Facial Surgery are available to me? This patient underwent both repair of the ptosis (drooping upper lid margin) as well as excision of excess skin. Lower lid cosmetic surgery was also performed. After surgery, the brows are more relaxed since the forehead muscles are no longer recruited in order to keep the upper eyelids open.

Aging is, to a large degree, genetically determined. Environmental factors such as sun exposure, cigarette smoking, and underlying disease also have considerable influence.

The tendons that support the eyelids become loose with age. In addition, the muscles become thin and provide less support. Long-lasting results necessitate repair of the supporting structures of the eyelids by appropriate "tightening" procedures. A glossary section is handy to look up terms which are defined within the text as well.

Editor's note: When is the optimum time to have surgery?
This decision is extremely personal but is basically determined
*after consultation with the surgeon. **The longer the individual***

waits to have restorative surgery, the more difficult time the surgeon will have reconstituting the normal anatomy and reversing of aged skin and other tissue changes. It is difficult to totally flatten "crepe paper" skin. Such skin, when pulled in one direction, will be distorted in another direction. The good news is that simple office procedures help to rejuvenate the face especially when combined with cosmetic eyelid surgery.

The vicious cycle of aging leads to redundant skin and tissues that are improved by surgery. The disturbances created by age are less difficult to reverse at an earlier age.

Section 2

PREOPERATIVE EXPERIENCE

CHAPTER 2

How Do I Select An Eyelid Surgeon?

The decision of how to select an eyelid surgeon may seem perplexing on the surface. However, once the consumer realizes that there are specialists in eyelid surgery, the decision becomes easier. Within ophthalmology, **ophthalmic plastic and reconstructive surgeons**, also known as **oculoplastic surgeons,** specialize in cosmetic and reconstructive eyelid surgery.

WHAT TYPES OF SURGEONS PERFORM EYELID SURGERY?

The consumer has the opportunity to select a physician from one of several medical disciplines. As stated in the Preface, the following types of doctors perform eyelid surgery:

*   *Oculoplastic surgeons (board-certified ophthalmologists)*
*   plastic surgeons
*   facial plastic surgeons, ear nose and throat surgeons (otolaryngologists)
*   dermatologists

Editor's note: Consumers may choose a board-certified oph-thalmologist who, like Dr. Mauriello, subspecializes in eyelid surgery (and develops special surgical techniques).

WHO SHOULD PERFORM MY COSMETIC EYELID SURGERY?

The best kept secret is that ophthalmic plastic and reconstructive (oculo-plastic) surgeons) are board-certified in ophthalmology and dedicated to eyelid surgery.

The subspecialty of oculoplastic surgery is the field of medicine that deals specifically with surgery of the eyelid structures. Most importantly, because ophthalmic plastic and reconstructive surgeons are board certified oph-thalmologists, they have an intimate knowledge of the eye and its support-ing structures. Most people are simply not aware of this unique subspecialty. As of 2004, there are only about 400 such surgeons nationally. The American Society of Ophthalmic Plastic and Reconstructive Surgery (ASOPRS) is the subspecialty society composed of board certi-fied ophthalmologists who obtain specialized training and credential-ing in eyelid, tear duct, socket, and orbital surgery.

As of 2004, no subspecialty board certifications exist in ophthalmology for the various subspecialists:

· retinal specialists

· neuro-ophthalmologists

· glaucoma experts

· pediatric ophthalmologists

· ophthalmic plastic and reconstructive (oculoplastic) surgeons

ASOPRS Fellows such as Dr. Mauriello obtained specialized training in eyelid, tear duct socket and orbital surgery after receiving the the following training:

- one-year internship in medicine or surgery

- three to four year residency in ophthalmologythat leads to certification by the American Board of Ophthalmology

The ophthalmology residency typically follows four years of college, four years of medical school, and a one year medical internship. This residency includes surgery of the eye and eyelids. Surgeons subsequently apply for a two-year fellowship in Ophthalmic Plastic and Reconstructive Surgery approved by the American Society of Ophthalmic Plastic and Reconstructive Surgery (ASOPRS.org). After completing this training, ASOPRS candidates must pass an oral and written examination and write a thesis that is approved by the Thesis committee in order to gain membership into the Society as Fellows.

Increasingly, oculoplastic surgeons are concentrating their efforts on cosmetic surgery particularly of the eyelids, eyebrow, and mid-face (from the bone just below the eye, the inferior orbital rim, to the mouth). Indeed, landmark studies emanate from the ranks of oculoplastic surgery: Lucarelli MJ, Khwarg SI, Lemke BN, Kozel JS, Dortzbach RK. The anatomy of midfacial ptosis. 16:17-22, 2000. Some oculoplastic surgeons expand their expertise and perform cosmetic surgery including the lower face and neck and liposuction on other areas of the body such as the breast, hips, buttocks and thigh. Interestingly, the intumescent technique used for anesthesia during liposuction employs dilute concentrations of local anesthetic. This technique was developed by a dermatologist.

Botulinum toxin, type A (Botox®) was developed by an ophthalmologist, Dr. Alan Scott, a Pacific Medical Center, to straighten eyes with improper alignment in the late 1970's. The drug was later used by ophthalmologists to treat involuntary eyelid spasms. Presently, this drug is used by cosmetic surgeons in all disciplines to improve wrinkles in the face.

The consumer may be assured that surgeons who are board-certified ophthalmologists and members of the American Society of Ophthalmic PlasticSurgery (asoprs.org) have a certain level of expertise in performing eyelid surgery. Patients should query their surgeon about their particular field of interest and expertise.

> *Editor's note: Ophthalmologists were the first physicians to use lasers and to use hyaluronic acid within the eye. Restylane®, hyaluronic acid in a bound compound form, is used in the office to plump up wrinkles.*

WILL COSMETIC EYELIDS SURGERY CHANGE THE SHAPE OF MY EYE?
The simple answer is "no," as least not according to Dr. Mauriello's patients.

"Cosmetic" surgery is, in fact, "restorative" in that surgeons reverse the effects of sun damage and aging by surgical tightening of sagging skin, muscles, and fat without changing the shape of the eyes. In Dr. Mauriello's experience, people desire a natural appearance. Dr. Mauriello is guided by patient's old photographs that help him develop a surgical plan that is suited for the individual patient. He requests that patients bring old photographs to the initial examination.

SHOULD I HAVE AN EYEBROW LIFT?

While many surgeons presently favor procedures that surgically elevate the eyebrows, such procedures may be performed with small incisions in the scalp and facilitated by the use of endoscopes. However, it should be kept in mind that the eyebrow basically frames the entire face as well as the eyelids. Any change in contour and elevation of the eyebrows may change one's facial appearance. Eyebrow lifts, in Dr. Mauriello's opinion, are important when the brows are not symmetric and at the same level.

Why not perform eyebrow lifts:

- The shape of the eyebrow may change

- Eyebrow elevation also affects the upper eyelid fold but since the results of the eyebrow lift are not entirely predictable, both eyebrow and eyelid asymmetry may result.

- Studies show that the risks of small incision endoscopic lifts are similar to those of the old coronal ear to ear lifts including loss of scalp hairs, thick scars, numbness and sometimes pain in the forehead that may extend into the hairline

- Eyelid surgery combined with eyebrow surgery is lengthy and the final results unpredictable. It is difficult to assess the amount of the upper eyelid skin (skin fold) to remove at the time of surgery because the final brow position often changes with healing after surgery.

- Eyelid surgery alone, in Dr. Mauriello's experience, improves eyelid position without moving the eyebrows with great consistency.

Dr. Mauriello sometimes recommends office Botox to temporarily simulate an eyebrow lift. No patient has returned for a brow lift, yet the patients return for additional Botox treatments in the eyebrows, corners of the eyes, and the lower face and lips.

While aging causes significant brow descent, the aging eyelids themselves require signifcant rehabilitative eyelid surgery such that concomitant brow elevation may not only be unnecessary but also too time consuming to allow surgical correction during a single operation. Again, eyelid surgery alone is usually sufficient without brow surgery to improve a tired appearance.

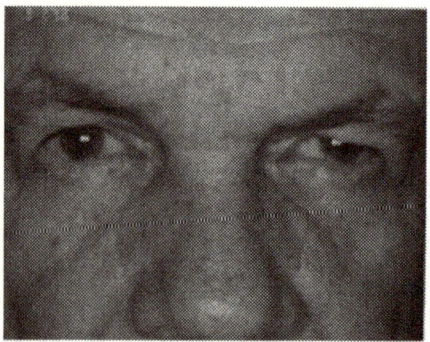   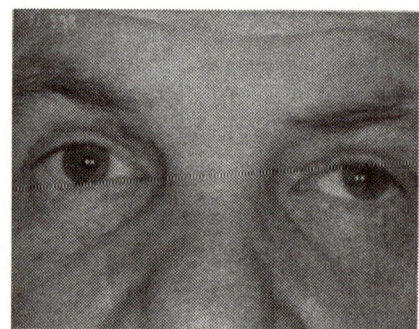

Figure 1   **Figure 2**

Elderly patient has significant excess upper eyelid skin and drooping eyebrows that affect vision (above, left). Note eyebrows are at same levels and appear symmetric. While this patient would benefit from a brow lift, he is quite happy to undergo a simple upper lid blepharoplasty or removal of excess upper eyelid skin through an upper eyelid skin incision without an eyebrow lift. After surgery (above, right), there is improved visual function since skin does not override the eyelid margin and block the pupil and obstruct vision.

In patients less than 55 years of age, brows rarely, if ever need to be elevated. Furthermore, when the eyebrow position is changed, the amount of skin that overhangs the eyelid crease, changes.

SHOULD I GO TO A SURGEON WHO ADVERTISES?

Increasingly doctors are advertising their talents. Some surgeons hire a publicist at great expense in order to obtain "brand name" recognition. Such physicians are often quoted in woman's magazines and may, in fact, provide free surgical care to writers and editors of the magazines. These surgeons may incur great expense and ultimately, if they are successful, have a high volume surgical practice. Volume is not a guarantee of quality although "practice" does tend to improve surgical results. The media has reported that some surgeons may perform surgery on radio and television personalities as well as magazine editors in order to win their favor and acclaim.

The best referral or advertising any surgeon can obtain is from a patient and also from another physician who has seen the surgeon's results over the years. Yet, advertising is one way that the individual doctor may make his (her) credentials, training, and expertise known to the public. A website is another excellent way. Advertising will probably increase in the future. Certainly, a patient should not be dissuaded from arranging a consultation with a surgeon who advertises.

The thrust of Dr. Mauriello's advertising is educational and it attempts to inform the public of the training and experience of ophthalmic plastic and reconstructive surgeons. This book is one form of advertising but its goal is also to educate.

WHO SHOULD PERFORM MY COSMETIC EYELID SURGERY?

Ophthalmic plastic and reconstructive surgeons(also known as oculo-plastic and oculofacial surgeons) are board-certified in ophthalmology and dedicated to eyelid surgery.

HOW DO I FIND AN OPHTHALMIC PLASTIC AND RECON-STRUCTIVE SURGEON?

The best way to find a surgeon is to contact the American Society of Ophthalmic Plastic and Reconstructive Surgery (222 South Westmonte Drive, Suite 101, Altamonte Springs, FL 32714 Phone—407-774-7880 Fax: 407-774-6440 or visit the website of the **AMERICAN SOCIETY OF OPHTHALMIC PLASTIC AND RECONSTRUCTIVE SURGERY:** www.asoprs.org. Dr. Mauriello agrees with Robert Goldwyn, MD, a plastic surgeon and Editor-in-Chief of Plastic and Reconstructive Surgery Journal. At the 28th Annual Scientific Symposium of the ASO-PRS on October 25th, 1997 in San Francisco, Dr. Goldwyn stated that surgical procedures should be performed by any surgeon who is able to benefit the patient regardless of background.

Surgeons of all disciplines should avoid a cookie cutter approach to cosmetic surgery and determine what, in fact, is bothering the patient. Ideally, you should ask the surgeon what complications may occur during the course of surgery. Ophthalmic plastic and reconstructive (oculoplastic) surgeons have training in ophthalmology and are able to handle virtually all complications. Significant pressure has been brought on the public to accept only a board-certified plastic surgeon for cosmetic surgery of all types. Such advertising may not be fully considerate of the patient's needs especially in the area of eyelid surgery.

Each patient should decide on a surgeon based on the following:

• credentials and background of the individual surgeon

- frequency that the surgeon has performed a given procedure
- informed consent that outlines the risks and benefits of surgery
- recommendations of other physicians and friends who have undergone the exact same procedure
- observation of before and after photographs of other patients
- office examination

However, as one reads this book it will become apparent that each procedure is so specialized that only after a personal consultation is the individual prospective patient able to best select a surgeon to perform their elective cosmetic eyelid procedure.

> *Editor's Note: The only way to make a final decision is to meet the doctor and ask him (her) to show you actual patient results and ask what is the particular field of expertise: liposuction, breast augmentation, face-lifts, or eyelid surgery.*

Frankly, no physician is able to comment directly on another physician's abilities unless he has operated with that physician and personally observed that surgeon's results over time. Indeed, it is rare for surgeons to be able to truly judge the work of a fellow surgeon.

WHAT QUESTIONS SHOULD I ASK IN THE CONSULTATION?

The average person does not have the time to do exhaustive research on any given surgeon. It is reasonable to ask the surgeon how many eyelid procedures the surgeon performs per week. An oculoplastic surgeon may perform 5 to 20 such surgeries a week. It is important to note that any eyelid surgery is cosmetic in the sense that asymmetry may be evident to even a casual observer. Simply, note a painting that is not hung straight on the wall. Its crookedness is usually apparent when one looks at the same wall from many feet away.

ASK TO VIEW SURGICAL RESULTS OF ACTUAL PATIENTS

Ask to see photographs of patients who have undergone surgery. In this manner, the prospective surgical candidate gains insight into the surgery, has fears allayed, and understands better the results of surgery. An educated patient is less anxious and more apt to comply with all post-operative recommendations of the surgeon.

> *Editor's Note: The purpose of this book is to answer many of the questions that patients ask prior to eyelid surgery and thereby to improve the entire surgical experience. While the principles outlined in the book apply specifically to eyelid surgery, they are helpful to any patient considering any type of cosmetic surgery.*

Additional questions will come to mind and others will be answered as you read the remaining text.

CHAPTER 3

What types of Cosmetic Eyelid Surgery are available to me?

Cosmetic eyelid surgery is better performed on individuals at a younger (35 to 55 years of age) rather than at an older age (over 55–60 years of age). With age, the support structure of the eyelid becomes weakened with age. Such changes need to be addressed at the time of cosmetic eyelid surgery. *Gravitational changes affect the tendons and structure of the eye. Sun-damaged and aged sagging skin contribute to this weakening. Loss of volume in the skin also contributes to the sagging.* Finally, changes in the underlying bone structure with age affect the eyelid appearance. Ultimately, the effects of age become permanent and contribute to themselves.

What causes the eyelids to age?
Sun damage and aging result in eyelid changes that are summarized in the following circular diagram.

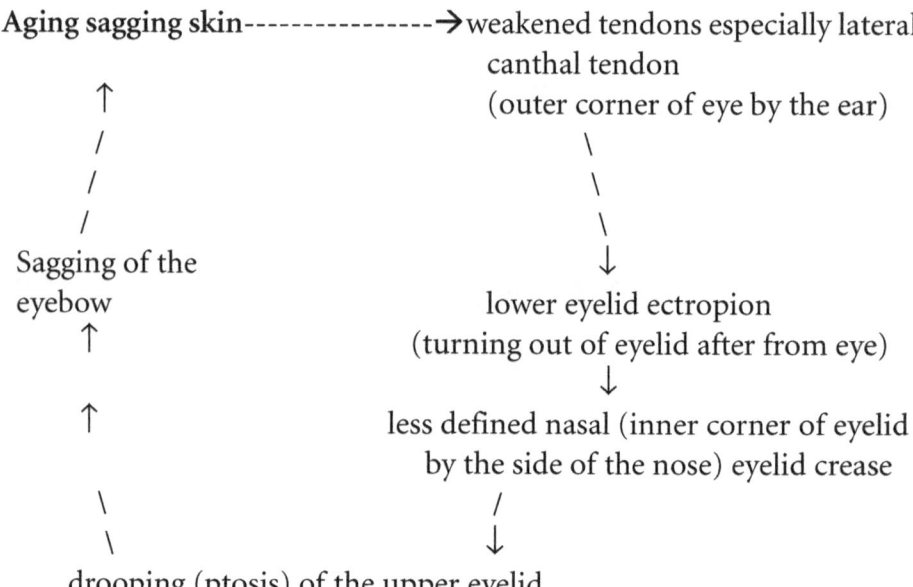

Aging sagging skin--------------→weakened tendons especially lateral
canthal tendon
(outer corner of eye by the ear)

Sagging of the
eyebow

lower eyelid ectropion
(turning out of eyelid after from eye)

less defined nasal (inner corner of eyelid
by the side of the nose) eyelid crease

drooping (ptosis) of the upper eyelid

With time, these changes are more difficult to *treat* than to *prevent* in their early stages. If the changes are severe enough, *reconstructive* and *restorative* **surgery** becomes increasingly more complex in order to re-attach weakened eyelid ligaments. Aesthetic eyelid surgery may not be performed without good underlying support, much as a house requires the proper foundation. The aged skin is similar to crepe paper and is unable to be flattened and smoothed. It has lost its hyaluronic acid and water content and, therefore, its volume. This volume depletion pro-duces increasingly thin and wrinkled skin.

> **Dr. Mauriello's observation:** *Patients may predict how their eyelids may look as they age by critically viewing the eyelids of the parent they resemble.*

This chapter provides an overview of eyelid aging and the various eyelids procedures and their purposes. Potential side-effects of the procedure are discussed to some extent but greater detail is considered in *Chapter*

4: Preoperative consultation—What I need to know about specific types of eyelid surgeries

Functional problems resulting from excess upper lid skin
Tearing and blurred vision: In patients with excess upper lid skin, an abnormal blink results with symptoms of dry eye due to evaporation.

> *Editor's Note: Excess skin creates heaviness which causes difficulty reading as well as dry eye symptoms including tearing, blurred vision and "grittiness." Sustained brow elevation to compensate for the eyelid droop or ptosis also affects the normal eyelid blink and lubricated state of the eye. Tearing may occur due to increased evaporation of components of the complex tear film due to incompleteness of each blink and a decreased number of blinks.*

The tear film is composed of mucin (mucous), aqueous (water), and lipid (oil). When the tear film is disrupted, the patient experiences, burning and itching. Any sustained elevation of the brow with abnormal blinking results in imbalance of the tear film and symptoms such as burning, itching, dryness, and foreign body sensation.

PROGRESSIVE SYMPTOMS OF DRY EYE
Burning and Itching
↓
Dryness
↓
Foreign body sensation
↓
Soreness
↓
Pain in the eye,
upper eyelid,
(rarely, the entire side of the face)

When the tear film is disrupted, the lacrimal gland may produce increased aqueous (watery tears) due to the imbalance of the various elements of the tears film. A watery tear (composed only of aqueous) may result. Over-the-counter topical lubricants may help restore the balance on a temporary basis in patients with excess skin overhanging the eyelid margin (dermatochalasis) and certainly in patients with ptosis (drooping of the eyelid margin). Patients with excess upper lid skin and true ptosis (drooping of the upper lid margin) may have increased symptoms.

Common causes of drooping upper eyelids from *levator aponeurotic dehiscence* (*separation of the levator muscle's tendon from its insertion*) include:

- excessive eye or eyelid rubbing, removal, insertion, and extensive manipulation of rigid contact lens especially hard contact lens and also soft lenses
- history of previous swollen eyelids from any cause
- previous eye or eyelid surgery

In certain patients with levator aponeurotic ptosis (*separation of the elevating eyelid muscle tendon from its insertion*) or the insertion is thinned, degenerated, stretched, and possibly infiltrated by fatty tissue. In some patients, evidence of drooping of the eyelid margin over the pupil (ptosis) may not be present when the patient is looking straight ahead but occurs only when reading.

With age, excess skin above the upper eyelid crease (dermatochalasis) and levator dehiscence (separation of the levator muscle tendon or aponeurosis from its insertion) may also occur.

Difficulty reading: Difficulty reading is often noted in patients with drooping upper eyelids. Individuals often tire after reading for a given period of time. Invariably if questioned carefully, patients comment that the vision improves when the eyelid is manually elevated. Some patients develop browache or headache since they constantly use their forehead musculature (frontalis muscle) to elevate the eyebrow and eyelids. Other patients mechanically elevate the involved eyelid(s) with their fingers after reading only a few minutes in order to see. Rarely, patients tape their eyelids up. More commonly, they tilt their head back in order to see. Such patients may develop neck pain.

What types of cosmetic eyelid surgeries are available to me?

Cosmetic eyelid surgery (Blepharoplasty—upper and lower eyelid)
Cosmetic eyelid surgery or blepharoplasty is the main procedure to rejuvenate the upper and lower lids and, in effect, the face.

• **Upper eyelid blepharoplasty** involves removing excess skin and fat prominence. In the most severe cases, the eyelid fold extends over the eyelashes and covers the eyelid margin.

Cosmetic upper lid surgery (Upper lid blepharoplasty): Upper blepharoplasty is performed through a skin incision that is concealed in the upper eyelid crease. A second incision is made above the eyelid crease in order to allow for excision of an appropriate amount of lax upper lid tissue. The wound is closed with a running suture that may removed 5 to 7 days after surgery. The eyelid crease is always formed where it naturally occurs.

> *Dr. Mauriello currently uses absorbable stitches that do not have to be removed. It is important not to remove too much upper lid tissue and thereby create a thin, skeletonized upper lid*

appearance. Bulging fat in the nasal portion of the upper lid needs to be removed. The crease must be reformed in the inner aspect of the eyelid where it is most visible.

The incision may be carried beyond the outer corner of the eye if excess skin or hooding occurs over the lateral or outer corner of the eye. Such overriding skin may become red, irritated, and itch.

The goal of blepharoplasty is to form a symmetric upper lid crease with the fellow eyelid and a symmetric fold of tissue that lies above the crease.

Editor's Note: Upper blepharoplasty is potentially a simple procedure with an excellent outcome. Yet, if performed too aggressively, that is, too much skin is excised, problems with dry eye may result from inability to blink normally. It is far better to have an undercorrection with residual upper lid skin than a minute overcorrection with minimally impaired decreased eyelid function and blinking and resultant uncomfortable, dry eyes. The oculoplastic surgeon because of his(her) knowledge of the eye is in an ideal position to assess the risk and treat even a transient dry eye after surgery.

BLEPHAROPTOSIS REPAIR: Should the upper eyelid margin droop or blepharoptosis repair be performed at the same time as the blepharoplasty?

The simple answer is "yes." Blepharoptosis is drooping of the eyelid margin. In individuals where the eyelid margin encroaches within 2 mm of the pupil (the cornea, that is, from iris to iris, is 10 mm in horizontal dimension), vision is affected. The eyelid margin is similar to a curtain over the eye and obstructs vision, much like a closed window shade limits the view outside a window. The upper lid blepharoplasty (removal of excess skin) is combined with a blepharoptosis repair (repair of a levator tendon or aponeurotic thinning or dehiscence). Sometimes excess skin weighs down the eyelid margin and creates a mechanical ptosis that repairs with a simple blepharoplasty.

Combined blepharoplasty and Blepharoptosis repair

Excess skin above the upper eyelid crease (dermatochalasis) and levator dehiscence (separation of the levator muscle tendon or aponeurosis from its insertion) may also occur. *Blepharoplasty and ptosis repair with the carbon dioxide laser* reduces the operative time so that support of the delicate eyelid structures can be strengthened and reconstructed at the time of blepharoplasty. The laser allows the surgeon to operate without time-consuming cauterization of tiny blood vessels throughout the procedure. The very difficult surgical positioning of the upper eyelid margin is facilitated by use of the laser. The laser induces less swelling as compared to the increased swelling that may accompany conventional incisional surgery with a cold knife. Judging eyelid position during surgery is, therefore, facilitated by use of the laser.

The patient has a tired appearance.

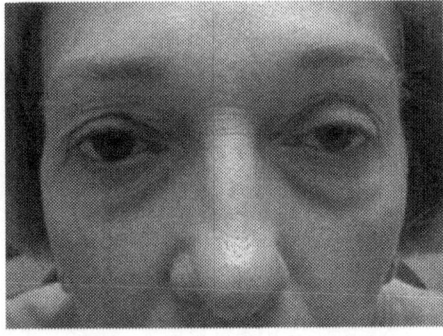
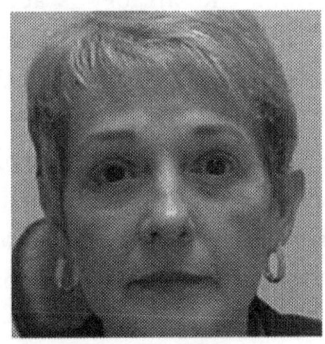

BEFORE   **AFTER SURGERY**

The patient photographed (above left) has a moderate amount of excess skin of the upper eyelid known as dermatochalasis) but also **blepharoptosis** (ptosis or drooping of the left upper eyelid). The left upper eyelid margin partially blocks the pupil and interferes with vision. The eyelid is like a window shade which blocks vision by covering the pupil.

The results are shown approximately 3 months after surgery. The eyes appear more open. Notice how the entire face appears rejuvenated since the:

- Eyes are open
- Upper cheek pads are elevated

Cosmetic lower lid surgery (Lower Blepharoplasty): Lower blepharoplasty rejuvenates the area from the lower eyelid margin down to mid-cheek area. It also serves to remove excess skin and bulging fat from below the eyelid margin down to the bone of the lower orbital rim (the bone just below the eyeball) through an incision that is just below the lash line across the lower eyelid.

Transconjunctival approach to lower eyelid blepharoplasty: If only fat is protruding, the surgery is accomplished without a skin incision. A conjunctival incision (the conjunctiva is the clear layer that "joins" the eyelid to the eyeball) is made on the inside of the lower eyelid. Since this approach does not violate the orbital septum, a thin fibrous layer that separates the eyelid from the orbit and its fat, the risk of causing lower eyelid pull down to cause scleral show is reduced. The transconjunctival approach is, therefore, better than the traditional blepharoplasty performed through a skin incision only (Refer to Chapter 1, Figures 9 and 10).

Dr. Mauriello's 3-step lower blepharoplasty technique: Excess skin appears as redundant folds of skin and/or wrinkles (rhytids). These so-called crow's feet extend outward from the outer corner of the eye. Blepharoplasty improves these static lines that are present when the individual is not smiling or animating the muscles in the face. Again, such lines are improved but not eliminated by upper and lower blepharoplasty as shown in the patient below.

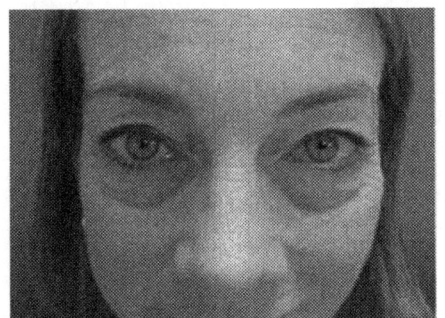

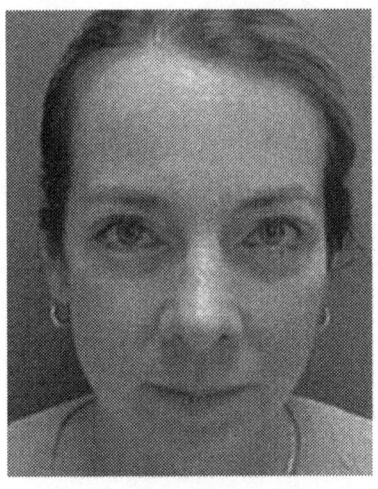

BEFORE   AFTER 4 LID COSMETIC
                         BLEPHAROPLASTY

Note cheek lift as evidenced by shortening of distance from the eyelid-cheek interface (above left) as compared to same distance 3 months after surgery (above right). Dr. Mauriello performs the lower lid incision through a small skin incision in the outer corner of each eye. The incision does not extend across the entire lower eyelid as is typically performed in the standard cosmetic lower blepharoplasty.

The orbital fat surrounds the eye and creates bulges under the thin eyelid skin, elevations, and shadows and circles under the eye. Bulging fat accentuates skin pigmentation as well to a certain extent. Skin pigmentation is a separate, more difficult problem that is only partially resolved by successful lower blepharoplasty. Specifically, removing such hills and valleys decreases the shadows. Dr. Mauriello's 3-step technique outlined below elevates the midface and thereby decreases the hollow that demarcates the lower lid from the sagging, aging midface. The pigment in the skin itself is not generally influenced by blepharoplasty. In fact, transient hemorrhage after surgery may temporarily and theoretically permanently add to the dark circles. Skin care with bleaching agents known as hydroquinones improves but does not entirely eliminate the pigmentation.

If there is excess skin as occurs in virtually all patients, surgery may be performed through a small skin incision just below the eyelid margin that extends in a laugh-line at the outer corner of the eye by the ear. The skin muscle flap is mobilized to help tighten the skin and elevate the cheek as well through this small incision. After the entire lower eyelid is undermined, the skin muscle flap is secured to the orbital rim at the outer corner of the eye. The size of the incision may be lengthened toward to nose depending on the degree of lower eyelid skin laxity.

Dr. Mauriello has created a procedure that tightens lower lid skin through a small incision in the outer corner of the eye (Mauriello JA: Three-step Technique to Lower Blepharoplasty. Ophthalm Plast Reconstruc Surg 2003 Nov;19(6):470-6.). The incision starts a few mm's from the lateral canthus and extends a few mm's beyond the lateral canthus (outer corner of the eye). This 3-step procedure removes the bulging fat, tightens the lower infrastructure, and finally creates a smaller template of the skin and muscle layer. The latter template forms a natural eyelid by tightening the back surface of the muscle with a carbon dioxide laser. Very little skin is removed. The stretched aged skin is tightened and placed back into position. Due to the thermal effects of the laser, the lower lid skin and muscle gradually tightens over 3 to 6 months to create a new natural, rejuvenated lower lid.

"V" Suture Horizontal eyelid tightening: Tightening of the lower can be difficult to perform consistently and effectively. Yet, it is absolutely critical to the success of the blepharoplasty procedure. The canthopexy/plasty is one of the most common procedures performed by ophthalmic plastic and reconstructive surgeons.

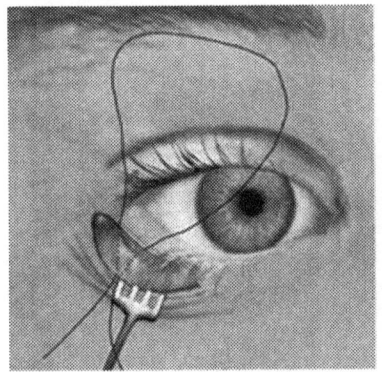 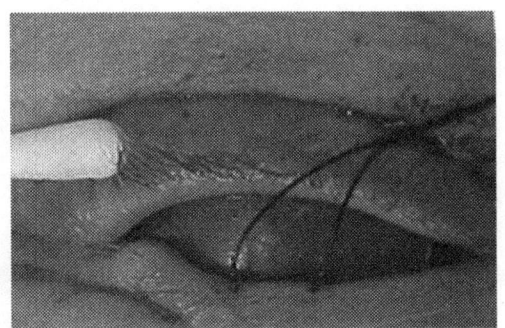

Dr. Mauriello's Commentary: Dr. Mauriello has developed a simple, single suture technique, a "v" suture (above left), that serves to tighten the lower eyelid. Notice the small pucker that forms when the sutured is tied to itself. The "wave" flattens with time on the intra-operative photograph (above right).

A loose clothesline will sag when only a few articles of clothing weigh it down. Tightening the lower eyelid stabilizes the lower eyelid do that scar tissue after cosmetic lower lid surgery does not pull down the lower eyelid. In addition, Dr. Mauriello uses steri-strips, a form of taping, to support the lower lid and the outer corner of the eye to enhance the effect.

In youth, there is a mongoloid (upward) slant to the outer corner of the eyes such that the outer corner of the eye or lateral canthus is 2 mm or 2/25 of an inch above the inner corner or medial canthus of the eye. With age, the lateral corner (canthus) descends and assumes an anti-mongoloid slant such that the outer corner of the eye is at the same level or below the level of the medial corner of the eye (medial canthus). Lower lid blepharoplasty should restore the upward slant of the outer corner of the eye.

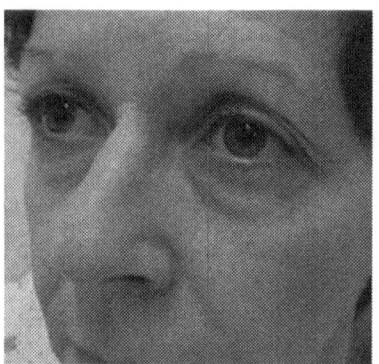 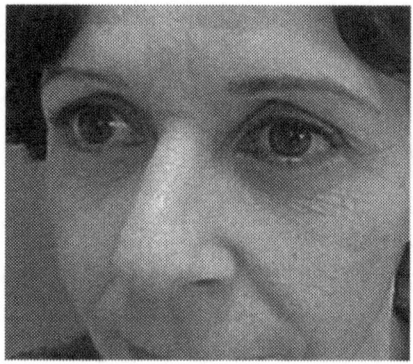

Note cheek depression prior to surgery with baggy lower lids (above left) as compared to cheek elevation (above right) and slightly upward slant of outer corners of both eyes 6 months after surgery.

The above patient underwent Dr. Mauriello's three-step technique:

• transconjunctival removal of fat

- "v" suture lower lid tightening
- skin muscle lower eyelid resuspension

After surgery (above right), oblique view shows improved appearance after lower lid blepharoplasty. No upper lid surgery was necessary.

> *Dr. Mauriello Commentary: The 3-step technique has been shown to elevate the upper cheek 3.5 mm. This elevation tends to improve the hollow between the lower eyelid and midface due to the sagging midface.*

Midface cheek lift: Using Dr. Mauriello's techniques, cheek lifts are performed through the same small lower eyelid incisions adjacent to the eyelids used to tighten the lower eyelid skin and muscle in a blepharoplasty. The sagging cheeks are elevated into their youthful position. The cheeks are lifted in a vector that is most importantly upward rather than outward towards the side of the upper face to provide a natural, unoperated appearance without creating a pulled, mask-like appearance.

Cutting instrumentation for cosmetic eyelid surgery: Surgery may be performed with carbon dioxide laser techniques to reduce surgical time. Because of the reduced surgical time and decreased swelling induced by combined cutting and cauterization of potentially bleeding vessels, the judgement aspect of the surgery is enhanced. This technique is, therefore, especially helpful in elderly patients with excessive tissues and for those individuals requiring multiple repairs including blepharoplasty combined with ptosis repair.

> *Dr. Mauriello Commentary: Most importantly, the laser tightens tissue and produces a smaller template of the previously distorted and stretched lower lid skin. This effect may be modulated for each patient by applying varying the amount of*

laser dissection. Traditional dissection with scissors may be necessary when less contraction of tissues is appropriate. In selected patients with a propensity for bleeding, the laser may be indispensable.

Blepharoplasty and other eyelid and facial procedures may also be accomplished with the traditional "cold knife" technique or with a variety of instruments that "cut" and "coagulate" at the same time including the Ellman Radiofrequency unit. The laser has definite advantages.

Eyebrow lift
Surgical elevation of the eyebrow is rarely necessary.
Individuals do not require brow lifts unless they truly wish to change the appearance of brows and face or have asymmetric brows. Brow elevation may increase the hollow between the lower eyebrow and upper eyelid crease. Any surgical brow lift will increase this hollow that is accentuated by aging with resultant descent of the eye and atrophy of fat.

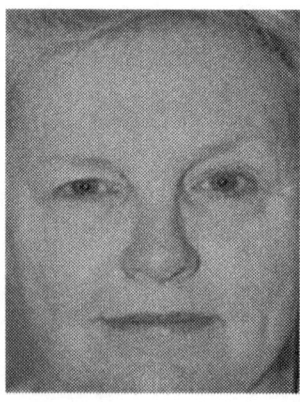
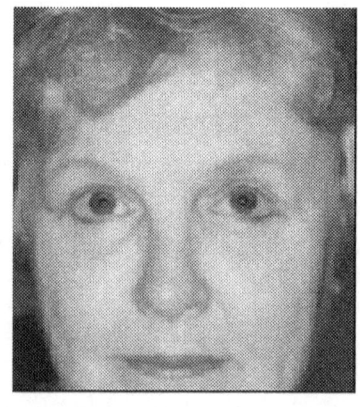

BEFORE   AFTER DIRECT BROW LIFT

The above patient has severe right-sided brow ptosis (droop of the eyebrow) with marked asymmetry. In such patients, repair of the eyebrow is necessary in order to create symmetric eyebrow position, the ultimate goal of all "cosmetic" surgery. After brow lift surgery, (above right), the right eye brow is restored to normal position. The incision was made directly above the brow.

Many surgeons presently favor eyebrow elevating procedures at the time of "routine cosmetic eyelid surgery. Such procedures may be performed with small incisions in the scalp and facilitated by the use of endoscopes. However, it should be kept in mind that the eyebrows basically frame the entire face as well as the eyelids. Any change in contour and elevation of the eyebrows may change appearance and create an operated appearance. Such changes have an entirely different appearance when viewed in three dimensions. (Please see **CHAPTER 2—How do I select an eyelid surgeon? Should I have an eyebrow lift?**)

As stated in chapter 2, the reasons for avoiding brow lifts except in patients with asymmetric eyebrows are listed below:

- The shape of the eyebrow may change
- Eyebrow elevation also affects the upper eyelid fold but since the results of the eyebrow lift are not entirely predictable, both eyebrow and eyelid asymmetry may result.
- Studies show that the risks of small incision endoscopic lifts are similar to those of the old coronal ear to ear lifts including loss of scalp hairs, thick scars, numbness and sometimes pain in the forehead that may extend into the hairline
- Eyelid surgery combined with eyebrow surgery is lengthy and the final results unpredictable. It is difficult to assess the amount of the upper eyelid skin (skin fold) to remove at the time of surgery

because the final brow position often changes with healing after surgery.

- Eyelid surgery alone in Dr. Mauriello's hands improves eyelid position without moving the eyebrows with great consistency.

> *Dr. Mauriello's Commentary: Brow lifts are rarely necessary for facial rejuvenation unless there is permanent brow weakness or brow asymmetry. Overelevation of the eyebrow just above the nose may produce a surprised look and create a hollow between the eyebrow and the upper lid which creates an elderly look. Most important, any change in the brow contour or shape may significantly change the patient's overall appearance since the brows outline the face and the eyelids.*

A brow lift, unlike a simple upper blepharoplasty, does not recreate an eyelid crease and potentially accentuates the hollow between the eyebrow and the upper eyelid. Most importantly, the final eyebrow position is now always predictable and the eyelid folds above the eyelid crease may, therefore, not appear symmetric. Symmetry is the key to successful eyelid surgery.

Finally, a study at Manhattan Eye and Ear hospital showed that the complications of endoscopic brow lift performed through small incisions in the scalp are very similar to those after more complicated brow lifts accomplished after a traditional coronal lift with a scalp incision that extends from ear to ear (Chiu ES. Baker DC. Endoscopic brow lift: a retrospective review of 628 consecutive cases over 5 years. *Plastic & Reconstructive Surgery*. 112(2):628-33; discussion 634-5, 2003).

> *Dr. Mauriello Commentary: When blepharoplasty is combined with a brow lift, there is a greater risk of post-operative*

dry eye than when either procedure is performed alone. Either upper eyelid surgery or a brow lift alone may adversely affect eyelid closure. For these reasons, there is a risk in combining eyebrow lift and upper blepharoplasty especially in patients with dry eye. That risk is exposure of the eye and possible dry eye that may necessitate additional treatment.

In the open technique, a strip of scalp is removed in order to elevate the eyebrow and forehead. In the open brow lift, a surprised look is more likely to result. The forehead increases in vertical height as the skin is elevated towards the top of the head. The procedure permanently weakens the brow frown and scowl lines.

> **Dr. Mauriello Commentary:** *Brow elevation may be simulated by office Botox injections. Any brow lift should be preceded by the these injections so that the patient and surgeon may determine if the cosmetic effect is appealing. No blepharoplasty patient in Dr. Mauriello's practice has requested a brow lift after Botox or after cosmetic eyelid surgery.*

Summary of why brow lift may not be optimal treatment:

- Brow elevation may increase the hollow between the lower eyebrow and upper eyelid crease and accentuate the loss of volume in the soft tissues of the face that are the hallmark of aging. Fat in the face is youthful.

- Because the eyebrow lift is generally supported 5 to 6 cm away from the eyebrow, the brow may descend with time. The exact amount of descent is variable. Unfortunately, any descent will affect the symmetry of the eyelid fold above the eyelid crease.

- The side effects of the endoscopic brow lift are similar to those of the traditional ear to ear coronal lift and include scars in the scalp with loss of sensation and hair

- Eyelid surgery alone creates a more symmetric upper lid fold than a brow lift. Moreover, the eyelid surgery creates an eyelid crease.

- In a patient with dry eye, the brow lift may unnecessarily contribute to eyelid closure problems. Eyelid surgery alone improves upper lid symmetry and removes heavy redundant upper lid tissue more predictable than a brow lift. The brow lift has a secondary effect on the eyelid. Eyelid surgery primarily affects the eyelid crease and the fold above the crease.

- Judicous use of Botox® can actually simulate a brow lift. In Dr. Mauriello's experience, patients do not request a brow lift after Botox injections because while the effects of Botox are temporary, they tend to be cumulative.

Suggested reading:

Mauriello JA. Editorial commentary on Blepharoplasty, Conventional and incisional laser techniques, Schiller JD and Bosniak S in Unfavorable Results of Eyelid and Lacrimal Surgery Prevention and Management, Chapter 1, 15-19. Mauriello JA (ed); Butterworth-Heinemann, Boston, Mass, 2000.

Mauriello JA. Editorial commentary on Incisional laser blepharoplasty and laser skin resurfacing, Khan JA in Unfavorable Results of Eyelid and Lacrimal Surgery Prevention and Management, Chapter 2, 53-54. Mauriello JA (ed); Butterworth-Heinemann, Boston, Mass, 2000.

Mauriello JA. Editorial commentary on Blepharoplasty and blepharoptosis surgery in Asians, Aguilar GL, Choo PH, Carter SR, Seiff SR,

Chapter 4, 68-70 in <u>Unfavorable Results of Eyelid and Lacrimal Surgery Prevention and Management</u>. Mauriello JA (ed); Butterworth-Heinemann, Boston, Mass, 2000.

Mauriello JA. Editorial commentary on Postblepharoplasty transeyelid subperiosteal midfacelift, Shorr S, Edelstein C, Balch KC, Shorr JK, Chapter 5, 131-132 in <u>Unfavorable Results of Eyelid and Lacrimal Surgery Prevention and Management</u>. Mauriello JA (ed); Butterworth-Heinemann, Boston, Mass, 2000.

Mauriello JA: Cosmetic eyelid surgery—The patient perspective—A retrospective review of 27 Patients: <u>Ophthalm Plast Reconstruc Surg</u> 19:320-322, 2003.

Mauriello JA: Three-step Technique to Lower Blepharoplasty. <u>Ophthalm Plast Reconstruc Surg</u> 2003 Nov;19(6):470-6.

Mauriello, JA. Preoperative evaluation of patients undergoing cosmetic blepharoplasty, Chapter 1, 1-17 in <u>Techniques of Cosmetic Eyelid Surgery: A case study approach</u>. Mauriello JA (ed): Lippincott Williams & Wilkins, Philadelphia, Pa. 2004.

Mauriello, JA. Upper and Lower Lid Blepharoplasty with combined blepharoptosis repair, Cahpter 2, 28-28 in <u>Techniques of Cosmetic Eyelid Surgery: A case study approach</u>. Mauriello JA (ed): Lippincott Williams & Wilkins, Philadelphia, Pa. 2004.

Mauriello, JA. Unfavorable results of cosmetic and upper and lower blepharoplasty, Chapter 3, pp. 67-96 in <u>Techniques of Cosmetic Eyelid Surgery: A case study approach</u>. Mauriello JA (ed): Lippincott Williams & Wilkins, Philadelphia, Pa. 2004.

CHAPTER 4

The Preoperative SURGICAL CONSULTATION—What do I need to know about specific types of eyelid surgeries? What are the roles of Botox® and Restylane office treatments for Facial Rejuvenation?

Undergoing cosmetic eyelid surgery is a bold endeavor. A "normal" person without disease requests that the surgeon improve his(her) appearance. The surgeon, in turn, states: "I can make you better." You need to have faith in your surgeon. This faith can only be earned after you are provided appropriate information about the planned cosmetic eyelid surgery. Ideally, cosmetic eyelid surgery should be performed by a surgeon who specializes in cosmetic eyelid surgery such as an ophthalmic plastic and reconstructive surgeon. Dr. Mauriello believes that board certified ophthalmologists with specialized training and credentialing (oculoplastic surgeons and members of the American Society of Ophthalmic Plastic and Reconstuctive Surgery, ASOPRS, www.aso-prs.org) are the ideal surgeons to perform any eyelid surgery because of their knowledge of the eyes and their specialization in eyelid surgery.

The preoperative consultation provides an opportunity for you to learn more about the surgical procedure (also, see Chapter 3, Surgical procedures), the possible complications of the various procedures, the usual surgical experience, and the post-surgical course. Educated patients will encounter less stress before, during, and after surgery. This chapter will help reinforce facts learned during your actual preoperative consultation.

PRE-SURGICAL EXAMINATION

Medical History
The physician always determines the chief complaint, that is, what is your primary concern about your eyelids' appearance and their function. The complaints may include:

- heaviness of the upper lids
- excess skin
- drooping of the upper lid margin
- dermatitis and itching induced by redundant upper lid skin
- bags under the eye
- sagging of the lower eyelid margin

The presence and duration of possible symptoms including tearing, mucous discharge, or blurred vision are also elicited. Tearing that clears after blinking suggests a problem in the tear film that may be due to inadequate lacrimal drainage or poor eyelid function. Again,

such complaints are routinely the province of the board certified ophthalmologist who specializes in eyelid and tear duct surgery, the ophthalmic plastic and reconstructive surgeon.

A history of itching, burning, or foreign body sensation with or without
tearing may reflect underlying dry eye, blepharitis, and eyelid dysfunction that may warrant treatment prior to cosmetic eyelid surgery. Your
surgeon is best able to treatment all such conditions.

It is important to bring old photographs to the examination. Old photographs are helpful in analyzing the progression and the nature of the
chief complaint. The nature of the chief complaint and other associated
symptoms are critical in determining whether the contemplated surgery is functional or cosmetic (See Table—Office Policy Regarding
Cosmetic Surgery). Photographs of the patient's mother, father, and
siblings may also be helpful.

A general review of the medical history is critical. In addition, a detailed
history of the outcome of any prior surgery is important. Specifically,
any problems that occurred from previous anesthesia should be discussed. In addition, bleeding or infection after previous surgery may
prove important in any cosmetic surgery contemplated.

PAST, FAMILY, SOCIAL HISTORY:

Smoking should ideally be stopped for one to two weeks prior to surgery, if possible, since smoking affects the blood supply to the face and
possibly the eyelids and may delay healing.

Alcohol intake should be minimized. Chronic long-term alcohol use
may be associated with liver disease and bleeding due to lack of clotting

factors normally produced in the liver. Similarly, chronic kidney disease may be associated with platelet abnormalities.

COSMETIC EYELID EXAMINATION

A complete examination that relates to eyelid function is performed by your surgeon. The form used in my office is provided below. Many of the examination are of a technical nature and are briefly described in parentheses following each entity. Detailed explanations when necessary are provided in the text below. All terms are available in the glossary and in **Chapter 1 Am I a candidate for eyelid rejuvenation? Eyelid Anatomy**

CHIEF COMPLAINT is the reason the individual wishes to have surgery. Is it the appearance of the upper lids, lower lids? Bulges through the skin, excess skin?

HISTORY OF PRESENT ILLNESS—
REVIEW OF SYSTEMS—PREVIOUS HISTORY OF PROBLEMS IN ANY OF THE FOLLOWING AREAS:

CHEST PAIN	_____YES	_____NO*
SHORTNESS OF BREATH	_____YES	_____NO*
OTHER:		
CONSTITUTIONAL SX'S	_____YES	_____NO*
(FEVER, WEIGHT LOSS)		
EARS	_____YES	_____NO*
CARDIOVASCULAR	_____YES	_____NO*
RESPIRATORY	_____YES	_____NO*
GASTROINTESTINAL	_____YES	_____NO*
MUSCULOSKELETAL	_____YES	_____NO*
INTEGUMENTARY		
(SKIN AND/OR BREAST)	_____YES	_____NO*

NEUROLOGIC   _____YES _____NO
PSYCHIATRIC   _____YES _____NO
ENDOCRINE   _____YES _____NO
HEMATOLOGIC/
LYMPHATIC   _____YES _____NO
ALLERGIC/
IMMUNOLOGIC   _____YES _____NO

PAST, FAMILY, AND/OR SOCIAL HISTORY (PFSH)
PAST HISTORY (ILLNESSES, OPERATIONS, INJURIES, TREAT-MENTS)
DIABETES???   _____YES
                        _____NO MEDICATION_____

HIGH BLOOD PRESSURE?   _____YES
                        _____NO MEDICATION_____
BLEEDING PROBLEMS   _____YES
                        _____NO TYPE_____
OTHER ILLNESS   _____YES _____NO
MEDICATION(S)   1._____   3._____
                2._____   4._____
PREVIOUS SURGERY: TYPE, YEAR
        1._____   3._____
        2._____   4._____

COMPLICATIONS OF SURGERY OR TO ANESTHESIA
        1._____   2._____

ALLERGIES TO MEDICATIONS
MEDICATION AND TYPE OF REACTION (RASH, ANAPHYLAXIS)
        1._____   3._____
        2._____   4._____

SOCIAL HISTORY
SMOKING _____*YES* _____*NO* *PACKS/DAY*_____
ALCOHOL _____*YES* _____*NO* *FREQUENCY—*
*ONCE A DAY*_____
*ONCE A WEEK*_____
*ONCE A MONTH*____

FAMILY HISTORY
DIABETES _____*YES* _____*NO*
HIGH BLOOD PRESSURE _____*YES* _____*NO*
CANCER _____*YES* _____*NO*
OTHER _____

EYELID AND OPHTHALMOLOGIC EXAMINATION (Form is abbreviated)

1. *VISION (Best Corrected)*
2. *GROSS VISUAL FIELD—Office test to determine if upper eyelid position affects vision*
3. *OCULAR MOTILITY (EVALUATES MOVEMENT AND ALIGNMENT OF BOTH EYES)*
4. *CONJUNCTIVAE*
   *Normal*_____ *Abnormal*_____

5. *EYELIDS—Photographs are taken of the eyelids and face*
   VERTICAL HEIGHT OF PALPEBRAL FISSURE (MM) _____
   (DISTANCE FROM THE UPPER EYELID TO THE LOWER EYELID MARGIN)

   UPPER EYELID MARGIN to UPPER EYELID CREASE DISTANCE (MM) _____
   DISTANCE FROM PUPIL TO THE UPPER AND LOWER EYELID MARGIN (MM) _____
   LEVATOR FUNCTION (MM) _____

LACRIMAL GLANDS may bulge through upper eyelids (outer corners) normally or in certain diseases—normal_____ abnormal_____

6. *PUPILS: SHAPE, SHAPE, AND RESPONSE TO LIGHT*
   (Pupillary response may indicate optic nerve disease)

7. *SLIT LAMP EXAMINATION*
   CORNEA—THE CORNEA IS EXAMINED FOR DISEASE AND FOR EVIDENCE OF DRY EYE
   TEAR FUNCTION
   TEAR MENISCUS _____
   (LEVEL OF TEAR FIILM VISIBLE AT LOWER EYELID MARGIN)

   DYE DISAPPEAR TEST_____ NORMAL _____ABNORMALITY (INDICATES WHETHER TEARS ARE NORMALLY DRAINING INTO THE LACRIMAL SYSTEM)

   SCHIRMER'S (5 MINUTES AFTER TOPICAL ANESTHETIC)_____ NORMAL _____ABNORMALITY (MEASURES AMOUNT IN TEARS IN TEAR FILM)

8. *LENS (OD, OS) CLARITY: _____YES _____NO*
   Diagnosis(es):_____ _____

   Plan(s)_____ _____

FURTHER EXPLANATION OF COSMETIC EYELID AND OPHTHALMOLOGIC EXAMINATION

The "best corrected vision" is the vision with corrective lenses. The movement of the eyes or ocular motility is assessed. The eye alignment in various fields of gaze is also determined and any double vision is noted.

Double vision is physiologic in that it normally occurs when any subject views a close object and sees distant objects double. Similarly, a single object viewed in the distance will make objects close up appear double. This phenomenon occurs because the eyes can only focus on a single object one at one time. Double vision may also result from the upper lid covering part of the pupil. Double vision due to a drooping upper eyelid margin or ptosis is temporarily improved by manually elevating the drooping lid and noting that the double vision immediately improves.

The presence of eyebrow droop or ptosis as well as eyebrow symmetry must be evaluated. Part of this evaluation includes the ability to elevate the eyebrows. Horizontal lines in the forehead as well as vertical wrinkles in the brow area particularly between the brows are photographed for the medical records. Prominent rims of bone above deep set eyes are also noted.

SLIT LAMP EVALUATION PRIOR TO SURGERY

An ophthalmologic slit lamp examination allows visualization of the optically clear structures of the eye. A beam of the slit lamp light traverses the eye tissues and the images are magnified. The examiner is able to determine the status and quality of the tear film. This evaluation is critical to the success of any eyelid surgery and should be performed by an experienced ophthalmologist prior to any eyelid surgery.

The normal tear film is complex and consists of three layers, an aqueous layer surrounding by an underlying mucin layer and overlying lipid layer that prevents evaporation. The tear film is maintained by proper eyelid function. The eyelid margins are examined for blepharitis or other abnormalities. Blepharitis is an inflammation of the eyelid margin. This inflammation may affect the tear film. A Schirmer's test or tear film test is performed to determine the quantity of tears.

A Schirmer's test is painless and may be performed comfortably after topical anesthetic eye drops are instilled into both eyes. The test takes a few minutes and provides valuable information that must be evaluated in conjunction with the slit lamp examination and complete medical history.

Various measurements are made from the eyelid crease to the upper eyelid margin. In addition, the distance from the center of the pupil in each eye to the upper eyelid margin is taken. The mm's of excursion of the upper eyelid are determined to reflect the function of the levator muscle (muscle mainly responsible for elevating the upper eyelid). In addition, the distance of the lower eyelid margin to the lower limbus (where the white meets the clear cornea at the lower most portion of the cornea).

Scleral show is a common after blepharoplasty and may cause symptoms of exposure.

> *Dr. Mauriello also measures the amount of upper lid skin from the upper eyelid margin to the lower brow hairs in the plane of the pupil perpendicular to the horizontal. Consideration is given to whether the patient plucks the eyebrow hairs.*

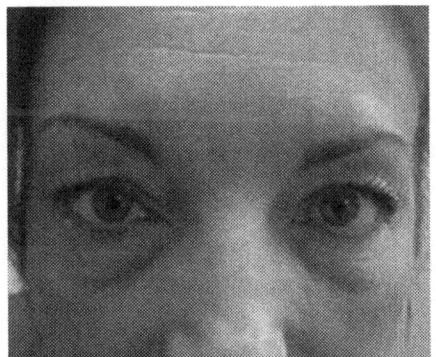
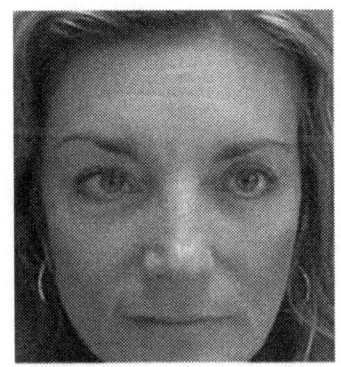

Figure 1
BEFORE

Figure 2
AFTER COSMETIC EYELID
SURGERY

Note improved and elevatd cheek position after lower blepharoplasty. Even when the upper eyelid margins are symmetric with respect to the pupils, excess upper eyelid tissue that overlaps the eyelid crease is apparent (Above, left). Note improved symmetry after 4-lid blepharoplasty (above, right).

The vertical (distance in mm's from upper to lower eyelid margin at its greatest vertical height) dimension of the opening between the upper and lower eyelids is measured and photographed. In addition, the horizontal dimension (distance in mm's from the medial corner of the eye by the nose, the medial commissure, to the outer corner of eye by the ear, the lateral commissure) of the eyelid apertures is measured. Any asymmetries are assessed. The elasticity of the lower eyelid is measured in order to determine whether the eyelid requires horizontal tightening at the time of surgery.

TEARING IS EVALUATED PRIOR TO SURGERY

If any tearing is present, the cornea is examined for dry spots or even subtle corneal breakdown due to dry eye or an "eyelid malposition."

> *Dr. Mauriello's commentary: Patients with the eyelid malposition known as entropion demonstrate that the eyelid margin turns in towards the eyeball and eyelashes irritate the eye (entropion). When the eyelid turns out away from the eyeball (ectropion), tearing results. All of these problems may be surgically corrected at the time of cosmetic blepharoplasty. Preoperative photographs are taken and are available at the time of surgery and help confirm all measurements.*

Selected patients with a cardiac or significant medical history should be examined by their physician prior to surgery. Such patients are given a medical consultation sheet and all patients are presented with a preoperative instruction sheet.

Functional visual loss results from either:

- upper lid excess skin that overhangs the eyelid margin. This condition is termed mechanical ptosis. If the eyelid margin descends due to the weight of the excess skin known as dermatochalasis, and partially covers the pupil
- true ptosis whereby the eyelid margin partially covers the pupil.

Visual Fields are performed in the ophthalmic plastic and reconstructive surgeon's office to demonstrate the effect of the upper eyelid eclipsing the field of vision above the midline. The test may then be repeated with the eyelid held open or taped. When the eyelid is taped open, the improved field of vision is evident for the purposes of medical insurance coverage. Whenever the upper eyelid is within 2 mm of the pupil, studies have shown that vision will be greatly influenced. A visual field while demanded by insurance companies is not necessary to document the field loss. Other functional problems associated with redundant skin include dermatitis or irritation.

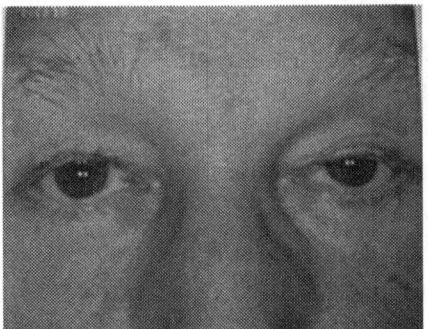 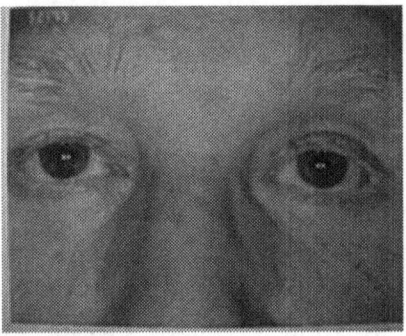

Figure 3
BEFORE SURGERY

Figure 4
AFTER SURGERY (PTOSIS SURGERY TO ELEVATE UPPER LIDS AND COSMETIC LOWER LID SURGERY

The patient photographed (above left) has true ptosis of the left upper eyelid after previous repair elsewhere. Note evidence of three separate left upper eyelid creases. Result (above right) after right and left upper lid ptosis repair and cosmetic lower lid blepharoplasty. Minimal upper lid blepharoplasty (removal of excess skin and bulging fat) was also performed in an effort to improve eyelid symmetry rather than for a truly functional reason. After surgery, the positions of upper eyelids are fairly symmetric with respect to the pupils. Moreover, the eyelid folds above the eyelid creases are also fairly symmetric.

General principles underlying all eyelid surgery
It is important for patients to realize that the eyelid is a highly, specialized structure that protects and has an intimate relationship with the
eye. The eyelid itself is thin and also delicate. Any abnormal eyelid function will affect the eye and corneal wetting and may cause symptoms
such as tearing, burning, itching, and foreign body sensation in the
involved eye. Any eyelid swelling or bleeding into the eyelid tissues during surgery will distort vision because the eyelid function is affected.

In the elderly especially because of dry eye, the tear film will be disrupted by any change in the upper eyelid position and any abnormal
eyelid blink. Eyelid dysfunction may temporarily decrease vision. The
eyelids prevent evaporation of tears and also help create a smooth surface to allow excellent vision. The upper eyelid is almost entirely
responsible for eyelid closure. The lower eyelid has little role.

> *Dr. Mauriello's commentary: Bruising of the eyelid tissues
> after surgery usually takes 7 to 10 days to resolve. Swelling gen-
> erally lasts 2 to 3 weeks. Patients tend to feel comfortable about
> their appearance by 10 to 14 days after surgery. At that time,
> makeup may be applied. Full physical activity may be resumed
> 18 days after surgery.*

Subtle scarring of the eyelid tissues takes several weeks to resolve. There
is a contractile phase of healing that starts approximately 2 months
after surgery last 3 to 4 months after surgery. During this period, the
eyelids may feel tight. The skin incisions may also become somewhat
reddened during the contractile phase.

> *Dr. Mauriello's commentary: When the contractile phase of
> healing diminishes the small incisions appear white and no
> longer have a "red" and tight appearance. The incision line*

reflects the scarring of deep eyelid structures that also relax with time.

No matter what surgical procedure is chosen, it is important to minimize the number of eyelid surgeries over the lifetime of any given individual. Multiple eyelid surgeries induce scarring that may adversely affect the normal blink and the tear film.

> **Dr. Mauriello's commentary:** *Even months after surgery, many imperfections will resolve as the tissues healing and remodel.*

INFORMED CONSENT

A crucial part to the success of any surgical procedure is the patient's understanding of the risks and benefits of each procedure. This understanding and acceptance leads to fewer surprises for the patient and ultimately a better experience for the patient. The risks and benefits are optimally carefully described to the patient's satisfaction in the preoperative consultation with the surgeon.

> **Dr. Mauriello's commentary:** *A detailed discussion of the risks and benefits of surgery are presented in some detail by your surgeon. Virtually, all events relating to surgery will produce a good outcome if treated appropriately especially if there is good rapport between you and your surgeon.*

Again, my belief is that cosmetic eyelid surgery is better performed at a younger (35 to 55 years of age) rather than at an older age (over 65 years). This aging is determined by your genetic make-up (look at your parents) and the amount of sun damage.

In addition, eyelid structural changes worsen with the increasing effects of gravity. These gravitational age-related changes are more difficult to treat than to prevent. In addition, loss of volume in the face due to loss of collagen and hyaluronic acid may be improved the skin care and tissue tightening modalties such as Thermage® as described in Section 2, *Chapter 3: What types of Cosmetic Eyelid Surgery are available to me?*

Type of anesthesia—Monitored Sedation
Eyelid surgery is performed under monitored sedation under the direct care of an anesthesiologist who may supervise a nurse anesthetist. During monitored sedation, the patient may receive supplemental oxygen in contrast to general anesthesia whereby patient's own breathing is done a mechanical respirator. Monitored sedation involves administration of both sedatives as well as narcotics by the intravenous route. These medications are often quickly reversible. However, since these drugs decrease breathing, a pulse oximeter monitors the amount of oxygen in the blood for the anesthesiologist. Sedation is augmented by local injections into the eyelids (local infiltrative anesthesia).

General Potential Risks of Cosmetic Eyelid, Blepharoptosis, and Other Eyelid and Facial Surgery
Every surgical procedure has risks and benefits. The individual undergoing the procedure should have knowledge of and the opportunity to ask questions about risks and benefits prior to surgery. This following section provides information about informed consent to the interested consumer at their leisure rather than in a relatively short surgical consultation or from a relatively uneducated friend. It does not replace the intimacy and one-on-one benefits of a pre-surgical consultation.

Potential complications of UPPER AND LOWER LID BLEPHARO-PLASTY (PTOSIS SURGERY) are listed below (and subsequently discussed in detail):

1. Eyelid and Deep Orbital Bleeding with possible loss of vision

2. Infection

3. Undercorrection, Overcorrection

4. Dry Eye

5. Persistent Eyelid and Eyeball Swelling

6. Blepharoplasty does not remove dark circles under the eye

7. Persistent tightness and Scarring of eyelids

8. Double vision (may be permanent)

9. Transient Numbness in the upper eyelid

10. Milia (tiny white bumps) may require additional treatment

11. Persistent crow's feet (lines in outer corner of eyes)

12. Consultation with additional specialists may rarely be necessary should an unusual problem develop

13. Additional surgery may be necessary

Each potential complication may be minimized in the following manner:

1. Eyelid and Deep Orbital Bleeding with possible loss of vision
In order to avoid potentially serious bleeding, all non-steroidal anti-inflammatory agents such as Motrin and Advil, should be stopped 5 days prior to surgery. All aspirin products and Vitamin E should be ideally stopped for 3 weeks prior to surgery. Please consult your prescribing physician before stopping any medications. Gingko, ginger, garlic, ginseng, fish oils, and certain Asian foods including mushrooms, should be avoided as well. Such substances affect platelet function and, therefore, may interfere with the normal blood clotting mechanism and result in bleeding and should be stopped 3 weeks prior to surgery. Of

prime importance is a previous history of bleeding after other surgeries such as dental work provides insight into potential bleeding problems.

Need to treat concomitant hypertension
The patient is informed that during surgery, the surgeon meticulously cauterizes or seals by heat all tiny blood vessels to avoid bleeding both at the time of and after surgery. This task is facilitated by the use of the carbon dioxide laser to cut and cauterize tissue. During surgery, blood pressure is monitored by the anesthetist. Elevation of the blood pressure may cause bleeding during or after surgery. Therefore, all blood pressure medication must be taken the day of surgery. Sedation helps to maintain the blood pressure at a normal and safe level. Similarly, any nausea is treated with medications after surgery in order to prevent vomiting which may also induce hemorrhage. After surgery, bending down whereby the patient's head is below the level of the heart or lifting may induce hemorrhage. It is important not to be active for the first 24 to 48 hours after surgery and to apply ice and keep the head elevated. Lifting any heavy objects must be avoided for the first 3 weeks after surgery.

Head elevation reduces swelling. There is no medical evidence that arnica, an herb, decreases bruising after any type of surgery. On a practical level, arnica is helpful but controlled studies have, to date, not supported the value of arnica unequivocally.

2. Infection vs. Allergy to Medication
The signs and symptoms of infection usually start gradually three to four days after surgery and not 1 or 2 days after surgery. In the initial 48-hour period after surgery, allergy to topical medication results in itching as the main symptom. Swelling and redness of the skin may accompany allergy or infection. The allergy may result from the medication or to the preservative.

Infection is heralded by decreased vision due to increased tearing and mucous discharge and also increased pain, swelling, and redness in the eyelid area. The vision clears for a few seconds after each blink. If any of these conditions are worsened as compared to their status the first day after surgery, the surgeon should be notified. Again, the first day of surgery is the baseline. Vision is checked at home on a daily basis. The newspaper is read with each eye individually covered.

The eye normally reacts to the surgery (planned injury) by mucous discharge from the conjunctiva (the outer covering of the eye over the white sclera) and tearing from the lacrimal gland. Again, tearing, swelling, pain, and mucous discharge assume greater significance when any of there parameters increases as compared to the previous day.

3. **Undercorrection, Overcorrection after Cosmetic eyelid surgery (Blepharoplasty)**
Others risks include undercorrection or removal of too little skin and protruding fat. Consideration for additional revisional surgery can only be made when the swelling decreases approximately 6 months after surgery. An early surgical intervention may only worsen the condition. It is not wise to pressure the surgeon to try to correct these problems earlier than 6 months and it is better to wait a year.

In the case of overcorrection, excision of too much skin (overcorrection) may prevent closure of the eyelids. Repair may require a skin graft to the upper eyelid. In this case, a new patch of skin may be cosmetically unacceptable. Removal of too much fat or constitute "bags" in the upper or lower eyelid will leave the individual with a hollow, skeletonized, unhealthy aged appearance. Undercorrection, that is, leaving slight amounts of excess skin or fat is always preferable since it is easier to take additional tissue away at a later date than to replace excised tissue.

Dr. Mauriello's commentary: To date, I have not had to revise a patient's surgery due to excision of too much tissue after a purely cosmetic eyelid surgery. Undercorrection is always preferable to excising too much skin. The latter almost invariably results in an operated appearance. More importantly, function may be adversely affected. Excess tissue may always be excised electively but it is much more difficult to replace tissues.

Crow's feet in the corner of the eyes may improve with blepharoplasty but are best treated with Botox injections. Smiling worsens the crow's feet.

Complications of Blepharoptosis (Drooping eyelid margin) repair
Variability of the eyelid position and double vision suggest myasthenia gravis although ptosis generally worsens at the end of the day due to fatigue. Myasthenia gravis which afflicted Aristotle Onassis is a neurologic condition. It may be limited to the eyes or affect the entire body musculature including the chest musculature and thereby breathing. Myasthenia is treated medically by a neurologist after appropriate diagnostic tests.

In the case of repair of drooping eyelid margins (blepharoptosis repair), undercorrection whereby the eyelid margin is just above the pupil is preferable to overcorrection. Since the eyelid is a complex but delicate structure, a single eyelid cannot undergo multiple procedures without affecting function. Each successive surgery increases the risk of additional scarring, a resultant poor blink of a thickened leathery eyelid, and aggravation of a dry eye. Cosmetic eyelid surgery does not change the underlying dryness of the eye but due to changes in the eyelid position and the completeness of the blink, a latent dry eye may become overtly dry. Because of the potential problems associated with repeat eyelid surgeries, ptosis revisions when necessary are best per-formed within 2 weeks of surgery (before scarring takes place) in approximately one in 20 blepharoptosis surgeries.

> **Dr. Mauriello's Commentary:** *After overcorrection, that is, the eyelid margin, is too high, corneal exposure may result with possible corneal breakdown, infection. If the patient is not fol-lowed by an ophthalmologist, even loss of the eye may result. Mild corneal exposure usually results from an incomplete blink, decreased frequency of blinking, and incomplete closure at bed-time. Mild problems often improve 2 to 3 weeks after surgery. Topical lubricating eye drops may intermittently blur vision since some drops are viscous. Patients are encouraged to blink with great frequency to clear the tear film and moisten the ocu-lar surface. In patients who have marked inability to close the eye at bedtime, ointments are used at bedtime. Dry eyes may persist for months and resolve without any permanent prob-lems. Such patients experience annoying tearing, increased blinking, blurred vision, and foreign body sensation due to poor lubrication of the ocular surface resulting from exposure of the eye due to inadequate upper eyelid function. In rare instances, permanent use of tears may be necessary. Other treatment modalities are outlined below.*

4. Dry Eye and Tearing

After cosmetic eyelid surgery, transient dry eye is common especially in patients with a history of dry eye. As stated above, dry eye is com-mon after an upper eyelid is elevated as in blepharoptosis repair (ele-vation of the eyelid margin but tightening the levator muscle of the upper eyelid). Such a repair will at least temporarily and rarely perma-nently exacerbate a dry eye. Increased evaporation of tears due to greater surface exposed after eyelid elevation results in symptoms of dry eye such as itching, burning, foreign body sensation, redness of the conjunctiva (the clear layer that covers the white protective coat of the eye, the sclera). In addition, some degree of usually temporary lagophthalmos (incomplete closure of the eyelids) may occur after surgery. Prolonged symptoms of dry eye occur in patients with severe dry eye but are certainly much more common in patients with overcorrections—that is, patients with shortage of upper and lower lid skin or in patients with marked scarring of the deeper eyelid structures.

> *Dr. Mauriello's Commentary: Patients with underlying dry eye may need to use topical lubricants on a hourly basis for weeks to months depending on the decreased frequency of blinking and the lack of full upper eyelid excursion. Eyelid closure is mostly a function of upper eyelid blinking. In the first two weeks after surgery, blinking is limited by mild discomfort. As a result, a decreased blink may lead to dry eye symptoms during this transition period. The symptoms of dry eye include itching, burning, grittiness, and foreign body sensation. The eye may appear red, inflamed, and there may be increased mucous and irritative tearing.*

Two weeks after surgery, the blinking is decreased by the tightness of the scar tissue which is beginning to form. The evolution of a scar is extremely slow. The tightness rarely may take six months to a year to completely decrease. In patients with borderline dry eye, the blink may decrease so that more of the ocular surface dries due to increased exposure and tearing results.

Dr. Mauriello has noted that dry eye after simple cosmetic eyelid surgery rarely, if ever induces, dry eye. However, any planned elevation of the upper eyelid margin such as ptosis repair may induce dry eye since more of the mucosa of the eye is exposed to drying.

Why does the eye sometimes tear when it is supposedly dry?
The tearing results from dry spots in the tear film that creates irritation and a watery abnormal tear. This tearing is similar to the effect that occurs when sand gets in the eye and the eye responds by secreting watery but nonlubricating, nonluxuriant tears. Corneal irritation is confirmed by superficial fluorescein staining on slit lamp examination in the ophthalmologist's or oculoplastic surgeon's office. Fluorescein is a special topical dye that attaches to areas of the cornea and conjunctiva where superficial layers of the outer lining or epithelium are missing. This orange dye fluoresces green when photo-stimulated by the cobalt blue colored light of the slit lamp. The conjunctiva (the clear layer over the white sclera) may become red due to dilated, inflamed blood vessels.

Slit lamp biomicroscopy (ophthalmic examination with special two (binocular) eyepieces affords a three dimensional view of the eye. Layers of the eyelid and transparent eye tissues such as cornea are seen with a light beam and high power.

> **Dr. Mauriello's Commentary:** *In all patients to date, no patient has required permanent use of tears after cosmetic eyelid surgery at a greater frequency as a result of surgery.*

The delicate nature of the eyelid tissues insures a long lasting result. The scar tissue induced by a single surgery is usually sufficient to maintain its cosmetic effect for a life-time.

*Eyelid cosmetic surgery, unlike face lifts, rarely needs to be repeated. The eyelid tissues have underlying muscle and each anatomic unit is supported by virtue of the cosmetic surgery itself. A **face lift** involves moving heavy tissues that do not include muscle. Heavy tissues mobilized by the face-lift include skin and underlying fat and fascia. Such tissues are heavier than*

those mobilized by cosmetic eyelid surgery. Moreover, in the face lift proce-
dure, such tissues are supported by sutures over a greater anatomic dis-
tance than is necessary for cosmetic eyelid surgery. For example, the facial
structures are dissected and supported to some extent by wounds in front of
and behind the ear. In contrast, during eyelid surgery, the skin-muscle
layer of the eyelid is supported only a few centimeters way from where the
eyelid structures are dissected. The eyelid is the only structure in the body
where muscle abuts skin and no intervening fat is evident between the skin
and the muscle.

A "touch-up" after blepharoplasty is rarely necessary in order to opti-
mize the surgical result. Such touch-ups are necessary in less than 5% of
cosmetic surgeries. Any early revision should be delayed at least 6
months but ideally a year after surgery to correct fine nuances. Surgical
repair in the immediate post-operative is almost entirely unwarranted.
The risks and benefits of revisional surgery must be carefully weighed
in each instance. Once the procedure is done, a "late" revision, years
later, may require only minimal surgery in order to rejuvenate the eyelids. No surgery lasts forever.

5.   Persistent Eyelid and Eyeball Swelling
While the black and blue in the skin generally is present for 1 to 3
weeks, eyelid and eyeball swelling usually last somewhat longer. Most
swelling has dissipated by 4 to 6 weeks. It may take 6 months or longer
for all traces of eyelid and facial swelling to resolve. Pre-existing cheek
swelling may be evident prior to surgery and may not improve after
surgery. Such edema may also persist for months. Increased pigmentation in the skin may accompany persistent eyelid edema but it occurs
especially after bruising of the skin. Bruising rarely takes months to
clear. Eyelid swelling may in part be precipitated by dryness in the eye
and associated eyelid inflammation.

Exacerbated Blepharitis (inflammation of the eyelid margin)
In addition, blepharitis is quite common with age and may be exacerbated by eyelid surgery especially in concert with underlying dry eye. Medical treatment of blepharitis including commercially available eyelid scrubs, topical antibiotics, warm compresses, and over-the-counter artificial tear preparations are helpful in treating this condition.

6. Dark circles under the skin
These circles are due in part to skin pigmentation and also by shadows created by depressions in the lower eyelid. Skin pigmentation present prior to surgery will not be improved by cosmetic eyelid surgery. Blepharoplasty does not remove skin pigmentation or melanin, the dark pigment in the skin that causes tanning. Depigmenting (lighten skin by decreasing melanin content) skin lotions such as hydroquinone or laser may be helpful.

> *Dr. Mauriello's Commentary: I have not yet referred any patient to a dermatologist for this treatment.*

By reducing the hills and valleys produced by prolapsing fat bags through the lower eyelid blepharoplasty using techniques, the skin appears smoother with less dark shadows. The shadows create an illusion of dark pigment which is improved by blepharoplasty.

7. Transient tightness and scarring of the skin and deeper structures
Scarring has various stages. One week after surgery, scarring is just beginning. With time, the incisions will become reddened due to contractile elements within the fibroblasts that make scar tissue (collagen). These contractile elements are necessary for the wound to mold and ultimately serve to maximize the eyelid function. Usually by 3 to 4 months, the thickened, red scar begins to flatten and turns white. The scar further remodels over a year.

Tightness of the skin rarely may last for up to one year after surgery, but in some patient the swelling may persist for several months. While a scar is mature after one year, scars tend to look better with each succeeding year.

Skin incisions may be carbon dioxide lasers sometimes cause permanent hypopigmentation of the skin or lightening of the skin due to decreased melanin pigment (the opposite of skin tanning). This tendency accentuates the eyelid scar. For this reason, during laser blepharoplasty, Dr. Mauriello does not make skin incisions with the laser unless the patient has lightly pigmented skin. In blacks, Asians, or patients of Mediterranean descent, laser skin incisions should be avoided. These pigmentations invariably decrease with time and normalize but it may take many months.

The incisions will gradually scar and initially feel thick but invariably loosen over time even without treatment. Massage with over-the-counter silicone gels and vitamin E creams may be helpful (**Section 5: SKIN CARE AND ADJUNCTIVE OFFICE PROCEDURES:** *Chapter 7: How do I take care of my skin after cosmetic eyelid surgery?* **Botox® and Restylane ® treatment after cosmetic eyelid surgery**). The upper eyelid scar is in the eyelid crease and is only noticed when the eye is closed. If the excision extends beyond the lateral canthus (corner of the eye by the ear), this lateral canthal area is more noticeable. The area may be covered by make-up usually 2 to 3 weeks after surgery. Scarring in the lower eyelid is present just below the lash line but may continue beyond the lateral canthus (corner of the eye by the ear) into the thicker skin of this region.

The skin in the upper and lower eyelids is thin while the skin of the medial and lateral canthus (skin around the corners of the eye by the nose, medially, and ear, laterally) form slightly more prominent scars than the eyelids. The skin of the nose and forehead forms thicker scars than the skin of the medial and lateral canthus. The cheek is less forgiving than the eyelids but forms less prominent scars that the skin of the nose and the forehead. All scars gradually improve with time. It may take up to 2 years for full improvement although most scarring is complete at 6 months.

Tendency to Scarring
(Listing in progression from tendency to form thinnest to thickest scars)
    Skin of the upper and lower eyelid
    Skin of Medial canthus (skin of corner of eye adjacent to nose)
    and Lateral canthus (skin of corner of eye near ear)
    Skin of the cheek
    Skin of forehead and Nose

8. Double vision
Double vision after any eyelid surgery is rare and usually transient if it occurs. While other treatments including prism glasses or additional surgery of the extraocular muscles is theoretically possible, such cases are extremely rare. Extraocular muscles surround the eye and are responsible for movement of the eye. If the eyes do not have synchronous movement, double vision may result unless there is significant fusion to overcome the muscle imbalance. The muscle may become weak from inadvertent injection of anesthetic directly into the muscle around the eye or from scarring due to the adjacency of the muscles to the orbital fat which is manipulated or removed.

> *Dr. Mauriello's Commentary: I have not sent a patient for any additional eye muscle surgery. Again, in the rare instances when it is noted it usually improves in a few weeks.*

9. Transient Numbness in the upper eyelid

Patients rarely note decreased sensation in the upper lid when they put on makeup. This finding has always been noted in woman when they place makeup and has been transient.

10. Milia (tiny white bumps)

These bumps usually form along suture lines and may require additional office treatment by needling the tiny cysts to express the cyst contents.

11. Impossible to remove dynamic crow's feet and smile lines

Crow's feet are wrinkles in the outer corner of the eye that are more evident upon smiling or after any facial movements or animation. Such "dynamic" lines do not decrease after blepharoplasty. Such wrinkles are best treated with Botox® (see *Chapter 4: Preoperative consultation—What I need to know about specific types of eyelid surgeries* **What are the roles of Botox® and Restylane® office treatments For Facial Rejuvenation?**). In contrast, static wrinkles present without facial animation may be improved to some degree. Thickened muscle under the lower eyelid evident when the patient smiles may be surgically removed. However, scarring of the muscle to overlying skin may produce less than desirable results.

12. Consultation with additional specialists may rarely be necessary should an unusual problem develop after surgery

Any unusual problem may require a second opinion from someone in the same or another field of expertise.

It should be understood that surgeons are always changing or modifying techniques in order to improve results. At times, a previous technique that yielded good results is abandoned for a modification that produces even better, more consistent results.

Dr. Mauriello's Commentary: Treatment of all complications after blepharoplasty is discussed in detail in *Chapter 7: How do I take care of my skin after cosmetic eyelid surgery?* Botox® and Restylane ® treatment after cosmetic eyelid surgery

COMPLICATIONS OF BROW LIFT

Brow asymmetry or contour anomalies
The main complication of brow lift is that a change in brow contour and position may alter the appearance of the entire face. For this reason, as stated above, brow surgery is rarely necessary unless you wish to change your appearance. In my practice, my indication for correction of brow droop or ptosis is asymmetric drooping of one brow. Even in older patients with excessive brow droop that affects both brows symmetrically due to the gravitational effects of aging, other eyelid structure are often drooping and require even greater surgical attention. It is simply too time-consuming during surgery to correct all four lids and then separately correct the brow. In addition, elevating the brow also affects the amount of skin to be excised in the upper eyelid. In my experience, the excision of excess skin in the upper eyelid is more precise and more long-lasting than brow surgery.

The brow lift may be performed through an upper eyelid or blepharoplasty incision. I favor this approach since the operating room time is decreased. Alternatively, it may be performed through an open incision across the scalp from the top of each ear. Currently, endoscopic techniques may be performed through small scalp incisions within the hair-bearing skin or alternatively through horizontal forehead lines. The risks which may be transient or permanent are summarized below:

RISKS OF BROW LIFT

1. Seventh nerve damage rarely occurs which might result in varying degrees of facial weakness or paralysis of the muscles that elevate the brow or close the eye. This complication can be temporary or permanent.

2. Asymmetry of the eyebrows

3. As with all surgery, complications such as infection or bleeding can occur and on occasion require appropriate treatment

4. Fluid or blood may accumulate in the operative site which may require further treatment

5. Blistering, crusting, loss of skin with delayed wound healing occurs in areas where the skin has been pulled too tightly after skin is excised. Such risks increase with smoking.

6. Patches of numbness over the forehead and scalp may follow surgery

7. Scalp itching

8. Diffuse temporary or rarely permanent hair loss which is more likely around the incisions

9. Lumps or irregular scarring that may resolve over several months

10. Irritation or dryness of the eyes

Since the endoscopic technique is less extensive than the open technique, it is, therefore, more likely than the open technique to preserve sensation of the top of the scalp. The brow is undermined and then fixated. The tissues are visually through small incisions with the assistance of the endoscope. Titanium screws are popular but perhaps the best fixation is achieved by creating tunnels in the bone under the scalp

(Lorenc ZP: How I modified the endoscopic brow lift. *Aesthetic Surgery Journal.* 19:489-490, 1999).

> **Dr. Mauriello's commentary: RESULTS OF BROWLIFT SURGERY:** *In a study of 25 patients carefully followed for a minimum of one year after examined after endoscopic browlift, 25% of patients had small areas of loss of hair adjacent to the wounds and scarring and 15% had changes in sensation that were noted at one year (Swift RW, Nolan WB, Aston S, Basne A. Endoscopic brow lift: Objective results after 1 year. Aesthetic Surgery Journal, 1999; 19:287-292). These latter problems are lessened by making bone tunnels to secure sutures that raise the brow. This technique is an alternative to fixating the brows to screws that are placed in the skull. In this study, the medial brow by the nose was elevated the most (2.4 mm). There are 25.3 mm in an inch. The outer brow above the corner of the eye was elevated 2.1 mm, the second most. The least elevated portion of the brow was that portion tangential to the outside corner of the cornea or lateral corneoscleral limbus (where the watch-glass (cornea)and colored iris meet the white or sclera) and that portion was elevated (1.9 mm).*

After endoscopic brow lift in a series of patients reported by Swift et al, no patients had the surprised appearance. However, it is well accepted that the ideal shape of the female brow is such that its highest point is over the lateral brow by the ear (lateral slant). However, Swift et al note that after endoscopic brow lift the highest point is at the medial brow (the brow adjacent to the nose). This effect creates a flat brow or masculine appearing brow in which the medial portion (above the corner of the eye by the nose) is most elevated.

Dr. Mauriello's commentary: In the Swift study, the scowl lines (vertical lines between the eyebrows) were not effectively removed. These scowl lines are dependent on a muscle that causes the vertical lines, the corrugator muscle and may be improved through an upper eyelid blepharoplasty incision and through small eyebrow incisions. Botox is a remarkable but temporary treatment of these lines (See *Chapter 7: How do I take care of my skin after cosmetic eyelid surgery?* Botox® and Restylane ® treatment after cosmetic eyelid surgery)

The supraorbital nerve that affects sensation on the entire side of the head courses through this muscle. Endoscopic brow lift by Swift resulted in decreased sensation of the forehead and scalp in 3 of 20 patients (15%) one year after surgery. Again, these lines may be treated in the office with Botox injections with virtually no risk.

BROW-LIFT POPOLARITY HAS DECREASED: In a retrospective study of 628 endoscopic brow lift procedures performed by 21 New York plastic surgeons over a 5-year period (1997–2001) at Manhattan Eye Ear and Throat Hospital the number of endoscopic brow lifts declined 70% from 1997 to 2001 (Chiu ES. Baker DC. Endoscopic brow lift: a retrospective review of 628 consecutive cases over 5 years. *Plastic Reconstructive Surgery.* 112(2):628-33). Seventy percent of patients were satisfied with their results, 50 percent of the plastic surgeons were pleased with the long-term results (after more than 2 years of follow-up). Complications of endoscopic brow lift included alopecia (loss of hair), hairline changes, infected hardware, brow asymmetry requiring surgical revision, prolonged forehead/brow paresthesia, frontal branch nerve paralysis manifested by inability to raise the brow, and abnormal sensations in the scalp (scalp dysesthesias). These complications were similar to those resulting from open brow lifts (Refer to *Chapter 4—*

The Preoperative SURGICAL CONSULTATION—What do I need to know about specific types of eyelid surgeries?)

Of perhaps greater importance is that fact that 71% of the surgeons routinely administered botulinum toxin type A (Botox) within 6 months of the endoscopic brow lift procedure. The authors concluded:

- the number of endoscopic brow lifts decreased due to the fact that selection criteria for the ideal endoscopic brow lift patients are currently more limited

- endoscopic brow lift is ineffective in the majority of patients

- no single superior surgical procedure for brow ptosis management is presently available

COMPLICATIONS OF ENDOSCOPIC BROW LIFT:

Temporary or permanent loss of scalp and forehead sensation
Rarely, permanent loss of scalp and forehead sensation, itching, and loss of hairs may occur especially around the scalp incisions with the open technique as well the closed, endoscopic approach. In the Swift et al series, 5 of 20 patients (25%) had some small areas of loss of hair or scarring over the fixation sites.

Facial droop due to seventh nerve damage (similar to Bell's palsy)
The seventh nerve that supplies the muscles of the forehead may be damaged. While rare, the degree of facial weakness may be partial or complete and affects elevation of the brow or closure of the involved upper eyelid and result in dryness of the eye. Sometimes during the endoscopic-assisted forehead lift, the surgeon may recommend a standard\forehead incision (ear to ear incision across the top of the head or in front of the hairline).

Infection and special bleeding problem relating to site of surgery
As in all surgery, complications such as infection or bleeding can occur
and require appropriate treatment including possible additional surgery. Fluid or blood may accumulate in the operative sites that may
require removal by surgery, simple drainage, or aspiration with a needle
at the bedside. Delayed wound healing associated with breakdown of
skin as shown by blistering, crusting, or loss of skin may occur. This
effect on the blood supply is noted with increased frequency in patients
who smoke. In addition, irregular scarring may resolve over several
months

Changes in the brow shape may significantly change the facial expression. A surprised look may result from overcorrection where the brow is
too elevated especially after the open technique. In such cases, the eye
may dry or be irritated due to incomplete closure. These symptoms are
similar to those occurring with excision of too much skin in upper lid
blepharoplasty or overcorrection of the drooping upper eyelid margin
(blepharoptosis overcorrection). An angry look may occur especially
with undercorrection (droop of the brow just above the nasal area). A
hollowed, aged look may be worsened by brow elevation which may
serve to accentuate the space between the upper eyelid crease and the
eyebrow.

I personally find rare indications for brow lifts and have not performed
an endoscopic browlift to date (Refer to Chapter 2, Figures 1 and 2).

Potential Complications of Laser Skin Resurfacing

*Editorial note: I do not perform laser resurfacing but provide
the following complications that are well known to dermatologists and should prove useful to the reader. My 3-step technique
smoothes and tightens the skin without the use of laser resurfacing.*

Complications include infection which may be bacterial, fungal in type, or viral such as Herpes Simplex and Zoster (shingles). Prior to laser skin resurfacing, prophylactic antibiotics and antivirals are generally prescribed. Skin care may suggested and include topical retinoids, alpha-hydroxy acids, and lightening agents for 2 weeks prior to laser resurfacing. Scarring may result from previous administration of Acutane, an oral medication used to treat acne. Such scarring is irreversible. Also irreversible is decreased pigment in the skin with possible demarcation lines between the untreated and treated areas. Increased brown skin pigmentation may be irregular but is virtually always transient but may last months. Complications may be transient or permanent.

Complications of carbon dioxide laser resurfacing

1. Redness, pinkness, or erythema of the skin that may last for several months and rarely up to two years

2. Facial crusting and pain usually for two weeks but may be prolonged,

3. Irregular scarring (especially if I have previously taken Acutane) which is more likely if previous scarring is present elsewhere on the body (I should avoid Acutane for at least one year prior to this procedure)

4. Increased skin pigmentation that may be localized or generalized Decreased skin pigmentation, that is, a light color, with possible lines of demarcation between the untreated and treated areas that may look different in color

5. Infection may be due to bacteria or fungus

6. Cold sores (fever blisters, Herpes Simplex of Herpes Zoster (shingles)

7. Changes in skin texture (feeling of skin) with possible depressions in the skin

8. Incomplete removal of damaged skin and/or wrinkles with residual wrinkles.

9. Persistent swelling

10. Pulling down or retraction of the lower eyelids

11. Injury to the eye (extremely rare)

12. Recurrences of wrinkles with time as aging continues

13. Reactivation of pre-existing acne or acne rosacea

14. Milia (tiny white bumps) may require additional treatment

15. New sensitivity to previously tolerated cosmetics

16. Consultation with additional specialists may rarely be necessary should an unusual problem develop

The most common complication of laser resurfacing is lightly pigmented appearance than may be permanent. Dark pigmentation is almost always temporary.

OFFICE PAYMENT POLICY FOR COSMETIC SURGERY

In general, payment for cosmetic surgery is received in advance of the surgical date. In individuals with a clearly functional problem such as ptosis where the upper eyelid margin or skin covers the pupil, the surgeon may elect to bill the insurance primarily for that part. At the time of a true upper lid ptosis repair, concomitant upper lid blepharoplasty, excision of skin or fat, for cosmetic reasons is the responsibility of the individual.

FUNCTIONAL UPPER EYELID SURGERY

There are definite criteria for functional as opposed to cosmetic surgery. If there is a visual problem, upper eyelid blepharoplasty or ptosis repair may be covered by the medical insurance policy.

Upper lid blepharoplasty is often deemed functional when eyelid skin overhangs the lashes and the patient experiences a definite heaviness of the upper lids. Patients will not difficulty reading due the weight of the upper eyelid skin. Dermatitis may result from redundant skin in the upper lid.

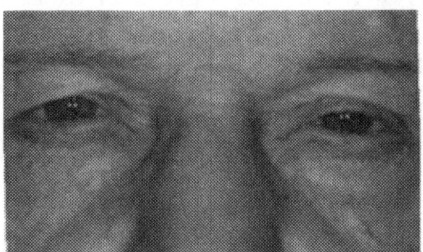
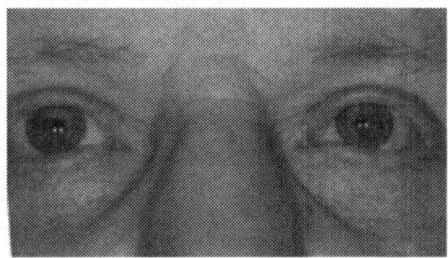

Figure 5
BEFORE

Figure 6
AFTER 4-LID SURGERY
INCLUDING REPAIR OF THE
DROOPING UPPER EYELIDS

(Above left) patient with functional right and left upper lid ptosis (drooping of eyelid margin) and excess skin (dermatochalasis). Right upper lid has considerable excess skin that overhangs the eyelid margin and affects vision. The left upper lid problem is mostly due to drooping of the eyelid margin or left upper eyelid ptosis. (Above right)

In case of ptosis when the marginal reflex distance (the distance from the center of the pupil to the upper eyelid margin) is 2 mm, of less, vision is affected. It is important for the patients not to unconsciously elevate the eyebrows when these measurements are made. The frontal muscle which elevates the eyebrow may falsely elevate the eyelid margins as well. Photographs may be taken in straight ahead gaze as well as oblique and direct views from the side (lateral) to show the eyelid skin overlapping the eyelid margin as well as the position of the eyelid margin from different angle.

Visual field test
Ophthalmologists perform computerized visual fields which objectively show interference with the superior visual fields (the field of vision above the midline) due to ptosis of the eyelid margin or excess skin overhanging the eyelid margin.

Lower eyelid surgery is rarely covered by insurance
Lower eyelids are virtually never covered by insurance unless there is eyelid laxity with significant tearing due to eyelid ectropion (loose lower eyelids that do not hug the globe). Such patients may experience tearing since the eyelid is turned away from the eye and the tears are not collected in the lacrimal drainage system. Rarely, the lower eyelids are so massively swollen that the lower eyelid skin hits the reading glasses. Ectropion or turning of the eyelid margin away from the eye results in tearing and exposure of the eye. These functional problems are almost always covered by insurance. Concomitant removal of prolapsed orbital fat (bags) is cosmetic and is not reimbursable.

Summary of eyelid procedures potentially reimbursed by Insurance
Upper eyelid blepharoplasty whereby eyelid skin overhangs the eyelid margin and when vision is affected, the fee is generally covered by insurance. All such determinations are ultimately made by the insurance company with the information provided by the doctor and the patient.

Upper lid ptosis repair whereby the eyelid margin partially obscures the visual axis and affects visual function is generally covered by insurance. *Lower cosmetic eyelid blepharoplasty* is not reimbursable. Significant **ectropion** of the lower eyelid that causes tearing is usually paid by insurance.

While the doctor provides information to your insurance, ultimately the insured is responsible for all inquiries. Again, medical insurance only covers functional surgery and no cosmetic element. If any of the above elements of surgery and the preoperative consultation are cosmetic and not covered, you are responsible for those elements not covered.

HMO's
I do not participate in any HMO's for several reasons. First, I believe they restrict medical care by trying to restrict access to expert consultants through "gatekeepers," so-called primary care physicians. In many cases, sometimes the best consultant for a particular patient's problems does not participate and, therefore, if a physician participates in a particular HMO, the patient cannot obtain a referral to that particular consultant. In the end, the patient suffers. The same problem applies to ordering tests. The bureaucratic red-tape in my opinion is so limiting that medical care is hampered. I do see patients in PPO's (preferred provider organizations) and POS's (point of service) since such plans do not directly intervene in the doctor patient relation. In such cases, the patient is responsible for coinsurance payments and deductibles and any part of my fee that is not covered. I do participate in Medicare. Medicare does not directly oversee every facet of specialty care as do most HMO's.

SURGICAL FACILITY

The surgery may be performed at an outpatient facility whether in a hospital, a freestanding surgery center, or in the office. I presently favor a hospital or freestanding facility rather than an office site because of greater medical equipment or personnel available should the patient require medical attention arise during the course of surgery.

FEES

Each fee should be enumerated by the doctor's office prior to surgery. Upper eyelid surgery generally is one hour and lower lid surgery is usually an hour but each surgery is individual and times vary. A nominal fee for photographs of the eyelids is necessary for medical care and such photographs are required by the medical insurance companies to obtain reimbursement for functional eyelid surgery. This fee may or may not be covered even if the surgery is functional. This fee is not covered by Medicare in New Jersey but is covered by many other medical insurance companies. The photographs help the insurance company determine whether the surgery is cosmetic or functional.

Similarly, visual fields demonstrate obstruction of the vision due to excess skin overhanging the eyelashes or due to true ptosis where the eyelid margin is within 2mm of the pupillary center. This test is generally but not always covered by insurance in advance of proposed functional surgery.

Again, insurance only covers functional surgery. If any of the above elements of surgery and the preoperative consultation are cosmetic and not covered, the patient is responsible for those elements not covered. Again, payment is due in advance of surgery for all surgery that is deemed cosmetic.

The individual may receive to statement to the effect that the:

> upper eyelid surgery is most likely:
>> functional and covered _____
>> cosmetic and noncovered_____
> lower eyelid surgery is most likely:
>> functional and covered _____
>> cosmetic and noncovered_____

In general, payment is expected prior to surgery.

The *facility fee* includes use of the operating room, nurses, equipment, and sutures. There is usually a separate fee for the services of an anesthesiologist/nurse anesthetist. Fees are generally based on an hourly rate.

General measures taken before cosmetic eyelid surgery include:

1. Ideally, avoid all smoking and alcoholic beverages for at least 2 weeks prior to and following surgery

2. Avoid all aspirin and Vitamin E for at least three weeks prior to and after surgery:
   (Other aspirin containing products—Ecotrin, Bufferin, Anacin, vitamin E, multivitamins, Alka-Seltzer, Bufferin, Coricidin, Darvon, Fiorinal, Dristan, Excedrin, Midol, Sine-Aid, Sine-Off, Percodan, Medipren)

Also, avoid gingko, garlic (supplements), ginseng, and fish oils (herbs may have pharmacological effects)

Non-steroidal anti-inflammatory agents (Advil, Motrin, or other anti-inflammatory for one week (to avoid blood thinning) prior to surgery
Take Tylenol
Check with your surgeon and your personal physician regarding Coumadin or Heparin

ALWAYS CHECK WITH YOUR PERSONAL PHYSICIAN REGARD-ING THE ABOVE RECOMMENDATIONS AND ABOUT RESUMING MEDICATIONS AND PLEASE NOTIFY DR. MAURIELLO

3. Do not eat or drink past midnight the night before surgery except for cardiac and anti-hypertensive medications with a sip of water

4. Please arrange transportation the day of surgery to and from the surgical facility and to have someone stay with you the night of surgery. Leave all jewelry and valuables should be left at home.

WHAT PROCEDURES ARE AVAILABLE IN THE DOCTOR'S OFFICE TO FOR FACIAL REJUVENATION?

BOTOX INJECTIONS TO SOFTEN WRINKLES

Botox (Allergan, Irvine, California) has been almost a miracle drug whose safety has been established since 1983 when it was first used as an experimental drug in children with crossed eyes.

About Dr. Mauriello's interest in Botox

In 1983, Dr. Mauriello visited Alan Scott, MD (Pacific Medical Center, San Francisco, California) who developed the use of botulinum toxin type A and demonstrated the effectiveness of botulinum toxin in the treatment of eyelid spasms in conditions known as blepharospasm and hemifacial spasm.

Dr. Mauriello was one of the first physicians to bring this treatment to the New York metropolitan area in 1983. An original investigator in National Institute of Health's study headed by Dr. Scott from 1983–1989, Dr. Mauriello was a consultant to the Committee of Ophthalmic Procedures Assessment of the American Academy of Ophthalmology from 1985–89 and was an invited to the Speaker's Bureau of Allergan (Botox®) Pharmaceutical Company, Irvine, California in 1997.

He also served on the Board of Medical Advisors of the Northern New Jersey Chapter of the national Benign Essential Blepharospasm Research Foundation from 1985–88. Dr. Mauriello participated in the combined NIH-National Blepharospasm Foundation Brainstorming Session in Washington, DC in late 2000. Since early 2000, he has been honored to serve as a Reviewer of the American Academy of Neurology's Therapeutics Assessment Subcommittee on Botulinum toxin therapy.

Basic Mechanism of Botuilnum toxin type A
Botulinum toxin type A temporarily weakens skeletal muscles. These injections soften facial wrinkles especially in the forehead between the eyebrows and in the corner of the eyes (crow's feet or laugh lines).

Botox office injections soften brow scowl and frown lines
The effect of cosmetic Botox injections is often enhanced by eyelid (blepharoplasty). They may raise asymmetric eyebrows. The single office treatments last between 3 to 6 months.

Botox injections temporarily improve forehead and brow frown and scowl lines by weakening the muscle responsible for such lines. It is also helps improve the horizontal lines on the side of nose at the level of the inner corners of the eyes. Weakening of the procerus muscle, a superficial muscle that brings the brow down when it contracts, helps reduce these lines.

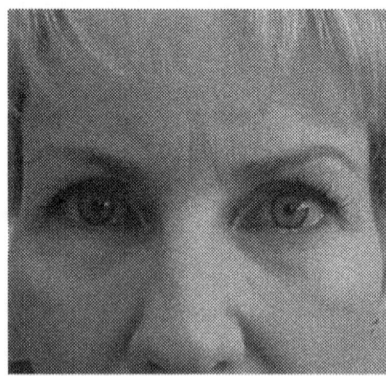   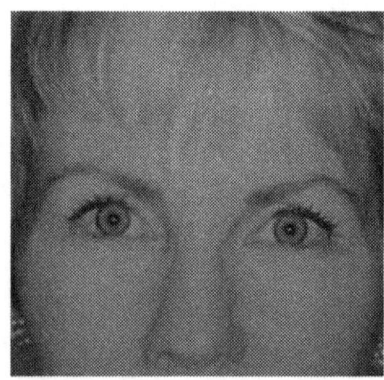

Figure 7
BEFORE

Figure 8
AFTER BROW BOTOX
INJECTIONS

Vertically and obliquely oriented lines between the eyebrows present a vexed and harried look. (above left). Office treatment with Botox results in a marked improvement (above right) and changed the patient's entire facial appearance. The eyes appear more open after the forehead treatment.

Botox office injections raise the asymmetrically lower eyebrow with improvement in brow scowl and frown lines

Botox selectively weakens the muscles around the eye that cause the brow to contract downward so the frontalis muscle (muscle that elevates the eyebrow) in the forehead is able to elevate the eyebrow and aging, sagging eyelid tissues with less effort. Static lines in the forehead may also be treated with Botox.

The crow's feet at the corners of the eyes may be improved especially the ones above the corner's of the eye. Too aggressive treatment of the crow's feet below the outer corner of the eye may affect the smile due to the muscle weakening effects of the Botox and rarely may affect the blink and result in dry eye. For these reasons, these treatments are optimally monitored by an ophthalmologist.

> *Dr. Mauriello's commentary: The ophthalmologist is in the best position to assess any effects of Botox on the eyelid and periorbital musculature that may ultimately effect the blink and the lubricated state of the eye.*

Botox diminishes lipstick lines and everts the lips to some extent

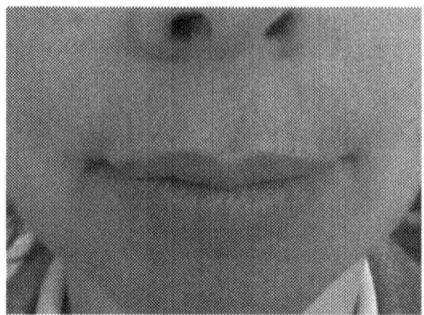

Figure 9
BEFORE

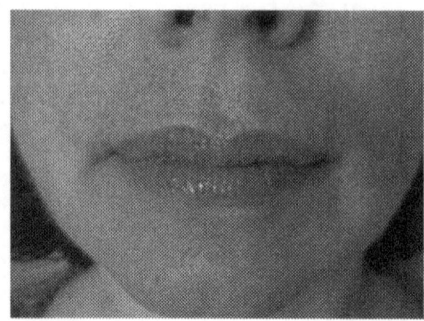

Figure 10
AFTER BOTOX

Lipsticks may be softened and the lips thickened for 2 to 3 months after Botox injections.

Facial cosmetic Botox provide relief without the permanent effects of surgery. The results may be cumulative. **The procedure may be done over your lunch-hour. The individual may drive to and from the office.**

RESTYLANE

Restylane is a "filler." Its effects probably last twice as long as collagen injections and no skin testing is necessary as with collagen. It is hyaluronic in a stable form that attracts water (hydrophilic). Hyaluronic acid is naturally occurring in all species and is found in humans in the vitreous (jelly) of the eye but also in the dermis of the skin. With age, the dermis of the skin loses hyaluronic acid and, therefore, water. The net effect is volume depletion of the skin. The cheeks of a baby are plump due, in part, to hyaluronic acid and the accompanying water it attracts. The effects of Botox may be enhanced and prolonged with the use of Restylane. *Restylane has virtually replaced collagen. The only advantage of collagen is that both forms of* bovine collagen (Zyderm I and II and

Zyplast collagen implant, McGhan Medical) usually do not cause as much bruising when injected. Human forms of collagen, CosmoDerm® and CosmoPlast®, are now available. They do not require prior skin testing as does traditional collagen but their effects do not last as long as Restylane®.

Fat injections may provide a more long lasting result but require more extensive surgery. The effects are not reversible and any result that is not optimal may represent a long term problem. Fat injections in the eyelids may cause a lumpiness that only responds to surgical excision.

LASER SKIN RESURFACING, CHEMICAL PEEL, DERMABRASION, THERMACOOL

> *Dr. Mauriello's Commentary: My patients do not request further skin tightening after undergoing blepharoplasty. The surgical techniques I use sufficiently tighten the skin that no laser or chemical peels are requested. They are encouraged to continue a regimen of skin care.* **Section 5: SKIN CARE AND ADJUNCTIVE OFFICE PROCEDURES: Chapter 7: How do I take care of my skin after cosmetic eyelid surgery? Botox® and Restylane ® treatment after cosmetic eyelid surgery**

The same changes that occur in the eyelids and orbital area also occur elsewhere in the face. Sagging skin and depressions in the aging face are due to decreased skin thickness and elasticity. Collagen thickens youthful skin but as it degenerates with age, it provides less support. There is gradual thinning of subcutaneous tissue including fat and loosening of the firm attachments of the skin to the underlying layers. In addition, gravitational descent of soft tissue occurs with the formation of skin folds along lines of skin adherence where the muscles of facial expression insert (Friedland JA, Simultaneous laser resurfacing with face lift: A safe alternative for facial rejuvenation. *Aesthetic Surgery Journal* 19:499, 1999).

Aging and sun-damaged skin may be treated with dermabrasion and chemical peels such as phenol for deep peels and trichloroacetic acids for more superficial peels. In general, the laser treatments have end points that are easier for the surgeon to identify than that of peels. The effect of the peel is dependent on the exact solution and its concentration, the length of time it contacts the skin, and the skin type and thickness.

Other skin treatments such as Retin A, glycolic acid, and topical Vitamin C are also useful and provide excellent benefits with almost no risk.

The office peel or microdermabrasion removes superficial (epidermal) layers and has minimal down time. The more invasive techniques provide more lasting effects but require varying amounts of post-operative care.

> ***Dr. Mauriello's Commentary:*** *Prevention is as important as treatment through an appropriate skin care regimen. Such a regimen is outlined in* **Section 5: SKIN CARE.** *It is important to incorporate a skin care regimen into your daily routine whether or not an individual ever undergoes cosmetic eyelid surgery.*

LASER SKIN RESURFACING: The short-pulsed carbon dioxide laser is used for skin resurfacing. It produces effects similar to the phenol peel. It produces thermal injury and the effects are perhaps monitored with greater precision, less risk, and side-effects. The carbon dioxide laser removes the outer layers of skin including the superficial papillary dermis without causing damage to the deeper reticular layers of the skin. When the process damages deeper layer of the skin, specifically the reticular dermis, permanent scarring may result. The laser has the effect of firming and tightening the dermis of the skin. All techniques whether chemical, mechanical, or laser initiated may result in permanent decreased pigmentation in the treated areas that may continue in the case of lasers two years after treatment. This prolonged duration of healing is not surprising the effects of accidental thermal burns may be seen for two years.

The greatest long-term complication of all these techniques is permanent loss of skin pigmentation. The neck area because of its lacks of hair follicles is subject to depigmentation but also to scarring after laser treatment. The cells emanating from the hair follicle reline the treated skin and result in scarring. Such a loss of pigment is increasingly greater in patients with dark skin as those of Mediterranean descent and Asians to even a greater extent. For this reason, the laser may be used for patients with a broader range of skin types than phenol peels.

Men are generally not candidates for laser resurfacing in particular because of the prolonged redness after treatment that may last weeks to months. Men will not find it socially acceptable to cover the erythema or redness with makeup. In addition, with recessed hairlines, the demarcation between the treated and untreated areas of the face will appear less pigmented or dark. The more darkly pigmented untreated may produce an unacceptable long term result. For this reason, a recessed hairline skin creates an artificial and unacceptable cosmetic effect after laser resurfacing. (Rosenbach A, Coblation: a new technique for skin resurfacing. *Aesthetic Surgery Journal*, 2000;20:81-83).

In general, skin found in the nasal and perioral areas tolerate a deeper treatment than the thin skin of the eyelid. The neck skin is thick but the risk of scarring is increased due to the lack of sebaceous units that are the source of cells that reline the damage skin surface after laser resurfacing.

Post-treatment infections are more common with laser resurfacing than the phenol peel for unknown reasons. Careful antibiotic and antifungal pretreatment reduce this risk significantly. Nonetheless, untreated or poorly treated infections may result in permanent scarring of the skin.

Carbon dioxide laser resurfacing is performed under local anesthesia with or without accompanying sedation with minimal discomfort. The initial healing process usually takes 7 to 10 days while redness may persist for several weeks but may last for several months to a year. Sun blocks are necessary for several months. The risks of scarring are quite real and must be considered. The other major drawback is the initial, sometimes painful healing phase that takes place during the first two weeks when the skin surface is relined. Significant redness of the face may persist for months to years. For these reasons, while this carbon dioxide laser resurfacing provides significant improvement, the postoperative course is not well tolerated and patients often would not opt for retreatment. The erbium-YAG laser combines ablation or superficial destruction without the heat effects of the short-pulsed carbon dioxide laser in order to reduce the sometimes difficult, postoperative healing period.

After such laser resurfacing, the laser wounds must be examined and cleansed by the physician every 24 to 48 hours with redness lasting from 2 to 3 months or longer as compared to the TCA peel where redness lasts 2 to 3 weeks. The partial thickness destruction of the skin (epidermis, the superficial layer of cells that cover the skin, and superficial (papillary) dermis heals by relining its surface (epithelialization) and formation of new collagen in the underlying dermis.

Skin resurfacing with the carbon dioxide and erbium ("weekend") laser improves skin tone, texture, and facial rhytids (wrinkles) and is particularly suited for the transconjunctival lower eyelid blepharoplasty that is performed without a skin incision. When performed on lower eyelids that are lax, the eyelid may retract due to skin contracture.

> **Dr. Mauriello's commentary:** *Less laser resurfacing procedures are being performed at this time due to the difficult post-operative recovery and skin depigmentation effects.*

Intense Pulsed Light
Intense pulsed light, an effective and safe method for skin rejuvenation, is optimum to remove pigmentation and small blood vessel markings known as telangiectasias. The technique reduces wrinkles to a lesser extent.

The ThermaCool or Thermalift (Thermage, Hayward, CA) Thermage tissue tightening performed in the office does not affect the superficial skin layers. Therefore, there is no effect on skin pigment. The radiofrequency device creates heat 2–3 mm below the skin's surface. Cryogen spray internally precools the electrode.

Treatment indications include wrinkle reduction, acne, skin rejuvenation, and various other aesthetic and therapeutic applications. The goal of this development program is to deliver an aesthetic or therapeutic benefit without burning the skin surface and without complications that require patient recovery time.

The radiofrequency (RF) energy uniformly heats the dermis while cooling and protecting the epidermis. It is designed to cause immediate collagen contraction followed by new collagen production which occurs over a period of time. As of 2004, the Thermage procedure is the most powerful method to tighten loose skin. *Long-term effects of this treatment modality are unknown, as of 2004.*

Each time treatment is delivered, there is an immediate cool sensation, followed by a brief hot sensation, and then a final cool sensation. An anesthetic cream applied one hour before the procedure numbs the surface of the skin to help make the treatment more comfortable.

> *Dr. Mauriello's commentary: With the advent of Botox® and longer lasting, natural fillers like Restylane, significant facial rejuvenation is possible with office procedures.* **Furthermore, Rejuvenation of the eyes and midface may be accomplished using Dr. Mauriello's special blepharoplasty techniques.** *Finally, tightening of the neck and jowl holds promise with new technologies such as Thermage. The key to this technology is that the skin surface is not broken down and there is no or little downtime and no pigment changes. Thermage-type technology may ultimately render the traditional face-lift unnecessary. The face lift that ultimately pulls skin from the midline of the neck to incisions in front of and behind the ear may not produce an optimal, anatomic result. Unless performed during the early stages of skin laxity, the traditional face lift tends to result in a pulled, operated appearance. Tissue tightening makes more sense at an earlier age than a traditional face lift at an older age.*

Suggested Readings

Mauriello JA: Blepharospasm, Meige syndrome, and hemi-facial spasm: treatment with botulinum toxin. Neurology 35: 1949–1500, 1985.

Mauriello, JA, Coniaris, Haupt E: Use of botulinum toxin in the treatment of one hundred patients with facial dyskinesias. Ophthalmology 94:976-79, 1987.

Mauriello JA, Aljian JA: Natural history of the treatment of facial dyskinesias with botulinum toxin: A study of 50 consecutive patients over 7 years. British Journal Ophthalmology 75:737-739, 1991.

Mauriello JA et al. Treatment profile of 239 patients with blepharospasm and Meige syndrome over 11 years. Brit J Ophthalmol 80:1073-75, 1996.

Mauriello et al. Long-term enhancement of botulinum toxin injections by upper eyelid surgery in 14 patients with facial dyskinesias. Archives Otolaryngology-Head and Neck Surgery 125: 627-31, 1999.

Mauriello JA: Blepharospasm, Meige syndrome, and hemi-facial spasm: treatment with botulinum toxin. Neurology 35: 1949–1500, 1985.

Mauriello, JA, Coniaris, Haupt E: Use of botulinum toxin in the treatment of one hundred patients with facial dyskinesias. Ophthalmology 94:976-79, 1987.

Mauriello JA, Aljian JA: Natural history of the treatment of facial dyskinesias with botulinum toxin: A study of 50 consecutive patients over 7 years. British Journal Ophthalmology 75:737-739, 1991.

Mauriello JA et al. Treatment profile of 239 patients with blepharospasm and Meige syndrome over 11 years. Brit J Ophthalmol 80:1073-75, 1996.

Section 3

OPERATIVE EXPERIENCE

CHAPTER 5

Blepharoplasty Surgery— Day of Surgery What do I need to know the day of my eyelid surgery?

Over the period of several years, Dr. Mauriello has canvassed a series of patients who had cosmetic eyelid surgery. The data answers all questions that patients asked prior to surgery. This chapter reflects their collective experience and is presented in a narrative form.

What happens on the day of the eyelid surgery?
The day of surgery, you are driven to the surgical facility. The night before surgery, you must not eat or drink after midnight. After registering at the facility, you are interviewed by the anesthesiologist. It is important to review your medical history briefly with the anesthesiologist. You should re-iterate any allergy to medication, problems with any surgery in the past, cardiac and pulmonary history, and bleeding history. A history of mitral valve prolapse should be elicited since it may require a single dose of antibiotic therapy administered intravenously.

Similarly, patients with prosthetic implanted devices may require a single dose of antibiotic intravenously. Your surgeon will greet you before the surgery. You will always be apprehensive but you will be glad to see your surgeon.

Type of anesthesia—monitored sedation?—Generally, patients report little, if any, pain associated with surgery. The anesthesiologist administers intravenous sedative-like medications which allow you to breathe on your own. The anesthesiologist may supervise and be assisted by a nurse anesthetist. Tell the anesthesiologist everything about your medical history.

Nurses in the operating room

1. Scrub nurse
In the operating room, there will be a scrub nurse to directly assist your doctor while he performs the surgery. The scrub nurse remains sterile along with the surgeon throughout the procedure.

2. Circulating nurse
The circulating nurse obtains various instrumentations and suture materials for your surgeon. Along with the anesthesiologist, she will make sure you are comfortable on the operating room table and that your body is positioned appropriately for the surgery.

Usual Chain of events in the operating room

- The anesthesiologist will start an intravenous line in your arm and you will receive medications to relax you. Narcotics relieve pain. Neuroleptic pharmacological agents create a dissociative anesthesia that relaxes you and provides amnesia for the event. In addition, minor tranquilizers sedate and relax you.

• The surgeon usually makes surgical markings on your eyelids at the same the anesthesiologist begins administering medications. You may be asked to open and close your eyelids. Topical anesthetic eyes drops are placed in the eyes. The drops are similar to those used in the ophthalmologist's office to anesthetize the eye's surface in order to monitor intraocular pressure. They may burn the eyes for 10–15 seconds and, therefore, you will be asked to gently close your eyes. After you are sedated, your surgeon often places a protective corneoscleral lens to protect the eye. The lenses shield your eyes from the bright operating room lights.

If there is upper eyelid drooping or blepharoptosis, your surgeon may ask you to look up during the procedure in order to surgically elevate the upper eyelid. At this time, the scleral lenses are removed and the operating room lights are dimmed in order to assess eyelid position. After the eyelids position is completed, you are sedated again in order to complete the upper eyelid surgery and cosmetic upper lid blepharoplasty.

The lower eyelid blepharoplasty is generally performed after the upper eyelids are completed. During the lower eyelid procedure, you may feel gentle tugging on the orbital fat. At such points, if you are aware of discomfort, additional sedation may be given. Similarly, local anesthesia may be supplemented.

You may wake up at different points during the surgery. If you feel discomfort, you will be able to talk and ask for additional sedation by the anesthesiologist. Local injections into the eyelid tissues by your surgeon will augment the anesthetic effect. Many patients are quite comfortable and do not ask for additional medication. You will not always hear what is happening around you.

In general, you will feel little discomfort throughout the procedure.

Recovery room
In the recovery, ice will be applied to the eyelids. You will encounter bloody tears but no constant dripping of blood. Any further nausea or pain will be treated by your nurse in conjunction with the surgeon and anesthesiology team.

The patient's reactions to all aspects of the surgical experience are described in detail in **Section 6: PATIENT TESTIMONIALS: THE PATIENT'S PERSPECTIVE** *Chapter 8: What can I learn from other patients who have undergone surgery?*

Section 4

POST OPERATIVE EXPERIENCE

CHAPTER 6

How to Care for myself after cosmetic eyelid surgery

WHAT TO EXPECT

Your level of anxiety about undergoing eyelid surgery should be greatly reduced after reading the previous chapters on the office consultation prior to surgery and the events at the time of surgery. This chapter provides further details about the practical aspects of care after surgery.

Care after surgery (General points)

The eyelids are extremely vascular and this attribute enhances rapid healing and decreases the risk of infection. Hemorrhage and consequent discoloration of the subconjunctival space are common and do not cause any discomfort. The subconjunctival space is the potential space between the clear conjunctiva and white sclera that is continuous with the clear cornea, the "watch glass of the eye." (See **Chapter 1: Am I a candidate for eyelid rejuvenation? Eyelid Anatomy.**

Blood may be present in subconjunctival space between underlying white sclera and overlying clear conjunctiva. In some cases, the white sclera is covered by bright red blood and even thicker layers of maroon-colored of blood under the smooth glistening conjunctiva. Like the bruises in the eyelids and cheeks, resorption of the blood in the subconjunctival space takes 5 to 14 days and is hastened by local application of ice for first 4 days after surgery followed by warm compresses to promote blood flow to remove blood breakdown products. Again, the red appearance takes 2 weeks to dissipate.

Regardless of whether subconjunctival blood is present, ice packs (baggies containing ice cubes) are necessary to apply to the eyelids almost constantly for the first 48 hours after surgery.

Frozen peas compresses
Frozen peas mold to the eyelids and are light in weight and well tolerated. Several packets should be available to rotate in the freezer. Transfer them to zip lock bags to isolate them from other items in the freezer. Place a thin sterile gauze between the eyelid and the baggies of ice or the frozen peas to avoid wound contamination. Either frozen device may be substituted with 15 minutes on and 15 minutes off. After the first 48 hours, apply ice packs four times a day for 10–15 minutes.

Enlist assistance the first 48 hours after surgery
It is very helpful to enlist the assistance of another individual the first 48 hours after surgery and certainly the night of surgery, it is mandatory not to stay alone. Many people return to work at sedentary occupations within 3 to 4 days but each individual has different rates of healing. Rates of healing are unpredictable. While there is no evidence to date demonstrates that smokers have clinically different rates of eyelid healing than others, I recommend stopping all smoking for at least one week prior to surgery. Smokers are at risk for poor vascularization after a facelift. Sample post-operative instructions are presented below.

Do not bend or lift
Any exertion including bending, lifting, and straining in the bathroom may cause bleeding especially during the first 48 hours after surgery. Bending down to tie your shoes should be avoided for the first 48 hours.

SAMPLE POST-OPERATIVE INSTRUCTIONS

1. APPLY BAGS OF FROZEN PEAS OVER A STERILE GAUZE BETWEEN THE EYELID AND THE PEAS FOR 10–15 MINUTES EVERY HOUR WHILE AWAKE FOR THE FIRST 48 HOURS AND THEN FOUR TIMES A DAY FOR THE NEXT 2 DAYS

2. DO NOT BEND FOR THE FIRST 48 HOURS EVEN TO TIE YOUR SHOE OR LIFT FOR 3 WEEKS. LEANING YOUR HEAD FORWARD MAY CAUSE MILD BLEEDING. AVOID RUBBING YOUR EYES. PLEASE WASH YOUR HANDS BEFORE AND AFTER ADMINISTERING ANY MEDICATIONS.

3. USE HOT COMPRESSES FOUR TIMES A DAY FOR 5 MINUTES STARTING THE SIXTH DAY AFTER SURGERY (check temperature of water to avoid scalding the eyelid skin)

4. IF YOUR EYES STICK TOGETHER UPON AWAKENING, MOISTEN YOUR EYELIDS IN THE MORNING WITH A STERILE GAUZE SOAKED IN COOLED, BOILED WATER TO SEPARATE THE EYELIDS (test the water temperature to avoid eyelid skin scalding)

5. USE ANTIBIOTIC DROPS IN BOTH OPERATED EYES— INSTILL ONE DROP FOUR TIMES A DAY FOR ONE WEEK

AFTER SURGERY OR UNTIL THE EYE DROPS RUNS OUT (ONE DROP IS SUFFICIENT FOR EACH TREATMENT). DO NOT MANIPULATE EYELIDS

6. SHOWER BUT DO NOT GET YOUR HEAD WET IN THE SHOWER UNTIL YOUR 1ST POSTOPERATIVE VISIT. DO NOT ALLOW THE WATER TO FALL DIRECTLY ON THE EYE.

7. CALL DR. MAURIELLO IF THERE IS ANY INCREASED PAIN, MUCOUS DISCHARGE, BLEEDING, OR BLURRED VISION (CHECK VISION DAILY BY COVERING EACH EYE AND READING THE NEWSPAPER PRINT. IN ORDER TO CLEAR THE TEAR FILM, PLEASE BLINK)

8. CONTINUE ALL MEDICATIONS YOU WERE TAKING PRIOR TO SURGERY BUT RE-START ASPIRIN/COUMADIN IF THERE IS NO BLEEDING THE MORNING AFTER SURGERY. (PLEASE CONFIRM WITH YOUR MEDICAL DOCTOR). CONTINUE ALL TOPICAL GLAUCOMA MEDICATIONS.

PLEASE CALL THIS OFFICE IF YOU HAVE ANY QUESTIONS— (908) 608-1200

As stated above, after 4 days of applying ice to involved lids to constrict blood vessels and limit the amount of tissue damage. If there is no bleeding, hot compresses are applied to the eyelids after water is boiled and is allowed to cool on the sixth day. A hot towel is placed over a moistened sterile (4 by 4 inch) gauze in order to protect the wound from infection. This heat is applied every 1 minute for 4 to 5 minutes at least four times a day the first week after surgery. Heat promotes healing by increasing the blood supply to the area. The patient photographed in my office a week after surgery experienced moderate redness of the eyelid and brow.

These effects occurred because she was applying to hot a cloth after it was heated in a microwave oven. Fortunately, the redness or erythema was transient.

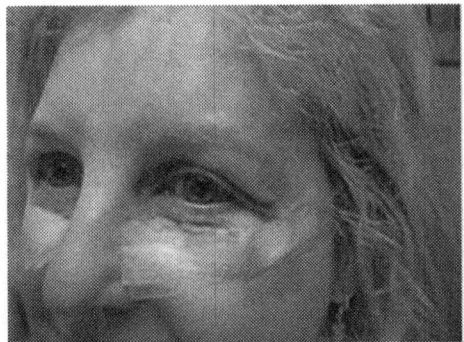

Figure 1—Avoid scalding skin with moist compress heated in microwave

The heat should not be so excessive as to scald the skin. Before applying any heat to the eyelid, test the temperature of the compress on the skin of the back of the hand first. The heat mimics the inflammatory response of the body that is designed to remove inflammatory debris from the surgically injured area.

COMMON OCCURRENCES AFTER EYELID SURGERY AND THEIR TREATMENT

Common occurrences after eyelid surgery are considered below along with their practical treatment. You may encounter all or none of the following after eyelid surgery.

Eyes Stuck Together, Blurry vision

If the vision is blurry, it is important to clear the tear film by frequent complete blinking. Gently cover each eye separately by cupping your hand but do not touch the eyelid wounds. Check the vision in each eye separately. Look in the mirror and observe whether the eyelashes are stuck together especially laterally the ear. Blinking may induce some discomfort the first few days after surgery. Tylenol (2 tablets every 4 hours while awake) should be taken for the first 3 to 6 days after surgery to increase the ability to blink frequently and more naturally.

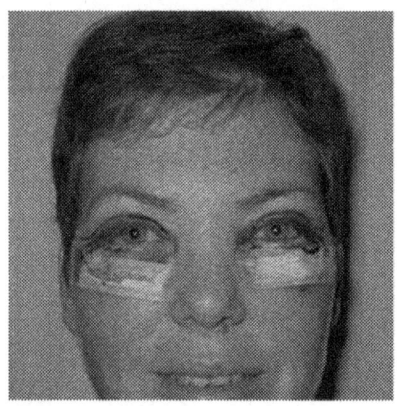

Figure 2:

DAY 3 AFTER SURGERY (above photograph)—Bruising of upper eyelids and swelling of lower eyelids is evident three days after 4-lid blepharoplasty. Steri-strips are kept in place on lower eyelids usually for one week to reduce swelling and to support eyelid in position until swelling decreases. Thickened upper lids blink poorly and over the counter topical tears are instilled in both eyes four times a day are necessary until swelling resolves.

Eyelid blinking is similar to the effect of windshield wipers that, like the eyelids, clear the windshield (cornea) with each wipe (blink). A complete blink such that the upper and lower eyelids meet is important. It is sometimes necessary to blink slowly analogous to the blink of a camel to enhance the tear film clearing effect.

If the eyelids are stuck together especially in the outer corners of the eye, a sterile 4 by 4 gauze soaked in boiled water is placed on the eyelids. The water is boiled since tap water may contain many contaminants. The water is allowed to cool, and a compress soaked in the water is placed over the involved eye repeatedly to soften any dried mucous. The upper and lower eyelashes are then gently separated. Topical antibiotic eye drops prescribed by your physician may also help to wipe out any mucous discharge or ointment which will blur the vision.

In general, eye ointments should be avoided because ointments only help to obstruct and blur vision. Eye drops rather than thick viscous ointment are used after surgery to avoid visual blurring. This recommendation was emphasized by a registered nurse who underwent eyelid surgery and was extremely upset because she believed she lost vision after blepharoplasty and did not know to gently irrigate the thick ointment out of the eyes. Rarely, a saline contact lens solution is necessary to wash out the eyes. Boiled water that is allowed to cool may be copiously applied to the involved eyelids as well. If the blurring persists, you should notify your surgeon immediately. If you have underlying dry eye, then tears more than four times a day may be necessary. In such frequent instillation of over-the-counter topical lubricants, tears without a preservative are usually less irritating to the eye. Drops have varying viscosities and the particular drop is determined by your surgeon based on slit lamp examination and severity of symptoms. Allergan Pharmaceuticals in 2004 offers the following products for dry eye from least viscous to most viscous:

    Refresh

    Refresh Plus

Refresh Liquigel
Refresh Celluvisc
Refresh PM Ointment

As stated above, the conjunctiva of the eye, the clear layer over the fibrous white sclera that supports the eyeball is billowed forward by tissue swelling (edema) or blood due to the surgical injury. The normally clear conjunctival surface is pushed forward by fluid and blood and becomes exposed. After surgery, tears that normally stay on this conjunctival surface run over its swollen surface and drip out of the eye. Increased blinking and topical over the counter tears will help to moisten its surface.

My patients are always provided my home phone number should they have any questions.

Eyes feels dry and are itching

On occasion, it is necessary to use topical lubricants (over-the-counter artificial tear preparations) for a few weeks and sometimes for several months after eyelid surgery. The need for tears may rarely be permanent. Patients with underlying dry eye that is diagnosed at the time of the preoperative consultation (see appropriate section) are told of this predisposition.

After any type of upper eyelid surgery, the eyelids do not blink fully or freely because they are thickened and swollen. Due to scar contracture that occurs from weeks to months after surgery, the eyelid blink is often incomplete. In all such circumstances, the tear film is not evenly distributed across the entire cornea.

Soreness of the eyes and the eyelids the first two weeks after surgery may affect the normal blink. The eyelid blink's completeness (amplitude), speed (rate), and number of blinks per minutes may be decreased. Since the normal blink is transiently diminished, the eye develops greater exposure, evaporation of tears, and relative dryness of the eyes and, of course, more symptoms. The symptoms include a progression from burning and itching, to a perception of dryness, soreness, and grittiness or foreign body sensation. The eyelid discomfort from the surgery may be exacerbated by the soreness of the upper eyelid that occurs in patients with dry eye who have not had prior surgery. The eye may tear, develop redness, and mucous discharge. The eyelids may become more swollen. Patients may simply elevate the lower eyelid in order to provide lubrication to the lower 1/3 of the cornea. This lower portion of the eye dries due to the temporarily hampered upper eyelid blink.

Dry may be aggravated by multiple eyelid surgeries in the past which diminish the completeness of the blink, speed, and number of blinks per minute

Usually, dry eye symptoms last a few days to 1–2 weeks but rarely the symptoms may persist for months. The symptoms in my experience always improve with time as the blink improves. The greater the scarring from any previous surgery, the longer it takes for symptoms to dissipate. Again, the blink is decreased due to eyelid swelling and discomfort especially for the first week after surgery. Tearing may also occur due to the dryness which again feels like there is sand or grittiness (foreign body sensation) in the eyes. Burning and itching usually precede the latter symptoms by hours or days. If untreated with topical lubricants, the eyes increasingly feel raw and sore. Intense itching may result from allergy to a topical medication or its preservative. If allergy is suspected, all topical eye medications should be stopped and your physician is contacted. The symptoms of allergy make take 2 to 3 days to subside after the medication is discontinued.

Again, the eye surface responds in only a few ways to dryness.

- The eye produces excessive watery abnormal, irritative tearing. Excess watery tears result from production of the aqueous tear film by the lacrimal gland and accessory lacrimal glands in a nonspecific response to the trauma of surgery. The accessory lacrimal glands are dispersed throughout the subconjunctival (space under the clear layer of conjunctiva) adjacent to the tarsus plate (the fibrous supportive plate of the upper and lower eyelids adjacent to the eyelid margin) and conjunctival fornices (spaces between eyeball and the upper and lower eyelids are also known as the upper and lower conjunctival cul de sacs).

- The normally transparent conjunctiva can become red and produce excess mucous from its goblet cell population. This mucin layer of the tear film is immediately adjacent to the eye. The lipid or fat layer is produced by the sebaceous glands of the eyelids, the meibomian glands. This outer layer of the tear film prevents evaporation of the middle, aqueous, or watery layer. Any imbalance in any component of the tear film produces symptoms of dry eye.

- Pain or changes in sensation occur and evolve from itching to burning to dryness to grittiness with foreign body sensation with the pain of "something sticking the eye."

- The dry eye may cause blurring since the patient is looking through a pool of water that sits on the lower eyelids and is not normally cleared by a complete blink. This pool of water particularly affects reading since the eyes are directed in a slightly downward position.

POOR EYELID BLINK AND DRY EYE SYNDROME

eyelid surgery-----> thick swollen leathery eyelid

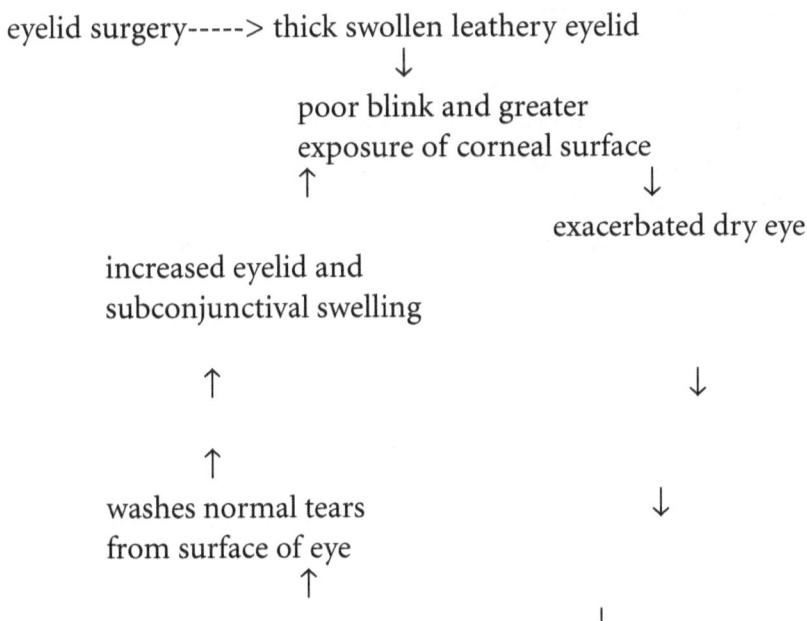

poor blink and greater
exposure of corneal surface

exacerbated dry eye

increased eyelid and
subconjunctival swelling

washes normal tears
from surface of eye

increased abnormal AQUEOUS
or water tears

Use of over-the-counter topical tears for dry eye
Topical tears of varying viscosity are used 3 to 4 times a day and are available without prescription from pharmacy but should not be used without the knowledge of your physician. In some patients, tears are necessary every hour to control the discomfort and secondary tearing. Rarely, an ointment is necessary. It is important to use topical tears without preservatives that are manufactured in small disposable vials. Drops with agents that constrict blood vessels should be avoided. Such agents initially whiten the eye by constricting the dilated, inflamed blood vessels but rebound dilation of the vessels invariably occurs.

Blanching conjunctival vessels may mask an infection or dry eye condition that requires medical treatment.

Tears without preservatives may be used in disposable small vials every hour while awake. Tears in a bottle generally have a preservative should be used no more than four times a day. The preservative is transient and dissolves. Rarely, such preservatives may be irritating to the eyes especially if used with increasing frequency and in the post-operative period. Avoid touching the eye with the eye drop dispenser at the time of eye drop administration. Refrigerated artificial tears are extremely soothing.

While dryness and itching may occur due to dry eye, the same symptoms may sometimes relate to allergy to topical antibiotics prescribed after eyelid surgery. For this reason, in patients with a history of multiple allergies to medications, topical antibiotics may not be prescribed by your physician.

Many patients prefer to use Refresh Plus (Allergan) at bedtime which is less viscous or thick than Celluvisc. Refresh (Allergan) eye drops are less viscous than Refresh Plus. Refresh, Refresh Plus, Refresh Liquigel, Celluvisc are all drops without preservatives. Rather than contained in a single-use small disposable vial, Refresh and the more viscous, Refresh Liquigel, are packaged in bottle-form that contains a preservative. The preservative dissolves upon eye contact and allows the lubricant to be stored in a multiuse bottle. Similarly, HypoTears Select (Ciba Vision) has a preservative, sodium perborate. This preservative is transformed transforms into water and oxygen and therefore minimizes any effect of the preservative on the eye. The advantage of these products is that they may be stored in a bottle and the preservative theoretically is not a factor upon eye contact.

Preservative free drops most often are packaged in disposable vials. It is important to avoid touching the eye with the tip of the vial if the seal is removed

Theratears (Advanced Vision Research) may be helpful especially when the mucin layer is deficient. Bion tears (Alcon) also helps to improve the mucin layer. Bion Tears contain bicarbonate and zinc. Research suggests that these ions may contribute to the stability of the superficial layer of the cornea, the epithelial layer, and its interface, the mucin layer of the tear film which bathes the cornea and conjunctival epithelium.

Genteal gel (Novartis pharmaceuticals) offers products as well. This soothing gel does not blur the vision as much as the ointments such as Refresh PM.

It is important to try one type of artificial lubricant for several days in order to find out by trial and error which drop provides the greatest relief. Ask your doctor.

If there is irritation in the eyes especially in the morning with the eyes crusting together, then the eyes may be open a crack at bedtime. At times, your spouse or significant other may check while you are sleeping with a flashlight during sleep to see if the eyes are open.

In such cases, you may use one of the more viscous drops such as Refresh Liquigel or Refresh Celluvisc (Carboxylmethylcellulose Sodium 1.0%, Allergan), rather than Refresh PM (Allergan) ointment because the ointment often blurs the vision upon awakening while Refresh PM is an ointment without a preservative. GenTeal gel (CibaVision) and certainly Refresh Liquigel ® may produce less blurring than other ointments.

Again, I prefer nonpreservative drops after surgery because any allergy to any additional chemicals in the tear preparation may only make the patient more uncomfortable. Allergy is heralded by itching, burning, and conjunctival redness ("pink eye") with a characteristic dry look to the reddened upper and lower eyelid skin. Itching is the hallmark symptom. The itching may mimic dry eye and your physician should be immediately contacted.

Topical cyclosporine (Restasis, Allergan) influence the inflammatory state of the eye show promise and are excellent for long-term treatment. Restasis may take up to 4 to 6 weeks to have an effect. Evaporation may cause a healthy eye to lose one-third of its moisture whereas a dry eye may lose as much of 3.4 of its tear to evaporation. Refresh Endura (Allergan) contains castor oil and helps retard evaporation by stabilizing the outer lipid layer of the tear film. It is the vehicle present in Restasis.

Practical Instillation of topical Tears (Lubricants)
The drops should be placed in the space between the upper and lower eyelids on the side of the nose. Always wash you hands before instilling medications and read the label prior to instilling. It is helpful to put medications in a Ziplock bag. It is only necessary that the drop hit the eyelashes. It will enter the eye by capillary action. Only one drop in the eye is necessary. More than one drop will not have any greater effect. The container of medication should not contact the eye to prevent direct injury to the eye and to avoid contamination of the bottle or vial of drops or tube of gel or ointment. It is helpful if the patient visualizes the tip of the eye drop container as it squeezed into the eye with the thumb and forefinger. The little finger may be held on the lower 1/3 of the nose as the fulcrum upon which to stabilize the hand to avoid direct contact with the eye.

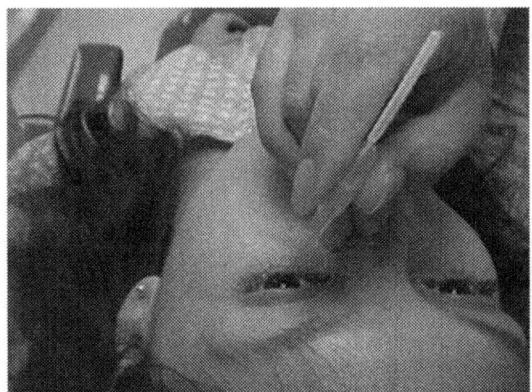

Figure 3
METHOD OF INSTILLING DROPS WHILE SUPINE

Drops are instilled without pulling eyelid down and are easiest to instill when lying down or semi-reclined.

In my experience, two patients have required topical tears for several months on an hourly basis after blepharoplasty surgery. This situation is unusual but is the result of delayed healing, tightness of the eyelids, and pre-existing dryness of the eyes. I have not treated a patient who permanently required tears any more after surgery than prior to surgery. Any pre-existing dry eye is diagnosed by your surgeon at the time of initial consultation. In some patients, the underlying dry eye may not produce symptoms until after surgery. The surgery does not cause the dryness but the decreased eyelid function due to the swollen, hemorrhagic eyelids allows the underlying, borderline dry eye to be manifest.

Use of punctal plugs for severe dry eye
After blepharoptosis repair (drooping eyelid margin), the upper eyelid margin is elevated and more of the ocular surface is exposed with resultant increased evaporation of tears. In patients with severe incapacitating

dry eye, consideration may be given to placing a punctal plug in the eyelid in the office. After a few drops of topical anesthetic are instilled into the eye, the tiny plugs are inserted into the lacrimal opening on the eyelid margin (near the nose) to limit drainage of tears. This procedure effectively retains tears to prevent dry eye. A simple office trial of an absorbable collagen plug which lasts a few days is usually predictive of the relief of symptoms that may occur with the more long-lasting silicone plugs. Such procedures are done by an ophthalmologist after a complete ophthalmologic examination. Plugs are rarely necessary after cosmetic surgery in my experience.

Medications predispose to dry eye
Rarely do dry eye symptoms last long enough to warrant stopping systemic medications and such medications may be reviewed by your surgeon. Oral flaxseed oil may be helpful in prolonged cases of dry eye. TheraTears Nutrition may be helpful. This product contains organic flaxseed oil (500mg), eicosapentaenoic acid (225mg), and docsahexaenoic acid (50mg) from fish oils. Oral Doxcycline may also be helpful along with eyelid hygiene and use of disposable Eyelid scrubs and hot compresses.

New medications FDA-approved to stimulate salivation have application for dry eye patients. Consult your oculoplastic surgeon or your ophthalmologist.

Pain after surgery
There is little pain associated with the surgery or with the healing stage most often. There may be mild soreness or discomfort. Tylenol only is necessary on the day of surgery.

Aspirin products and noncorticosteroidal (anti-inflammatory) agents such as Advil should be avoided. Should there be pain, bleeding, or blurred vision, your physician should be notified immediately at any time after surgery. Do not wait more than a few hours if symptoms persist. Generally, you will be able to drive safely 3 to 4 days after surgery. In this litigious society, however, patients are at risk driving with red swollen eyelids. Any accident may incur a lawsuit from another driver filed by a trial attorney. Your surgeon cannot take responsibility. Ultimately, the decision to drive is individual and is based on the degree of swelling and your overall response to the surgery.

Usually, you may resume vigorous activity after 18 days. You may take a shower the day after surgery and wash your hair. Do not allow water to continuously fall on the eyelids and face. Should the eyelids become wet, gently dry them with a towel. Wash the hair in the sink, bath tub, or at the beauty parlor. Some patients purchase swim goggles that shield the eyelids during surgery. Such goggles must be meticulously applied so that they do not mechanically injure the eyelid wounds. Show the goggles to your doctor.

DAILY SUMMARY OF MAJOR CHANGES IN EYELID AND PHYSICIAN RECOMMENDATIONS

Day One after Surgery

Swelling is almost always maximal the morning after surgery. Sometimes, anti-inflammatory agents (corticosteroids given intravenously the day of surgery and by mouth for 1 to 3 days after surgery) reduce swelling. The use of these agents can be particularly helpful. Corticosteroids, usually prescribed as prednisone, have multiple risks and should not be administered without the knowledge of your personal physician. Risks of oral corticosteroids include a small but increased propensity to hypertension, diabetes, infection, and even aseptic necrosis of the hip. The swelling in the eyelid region is always worse in the morning and decreases with the effects of gravity during the day when an upright position is maintained. The patient should avoid placing the heart below the head to decrease swelling and the risk of postoperative bleeding.

Check vision
The patient may check the vision daily by reading newspaper in each eye with the proper reading correction. The reading material is held 13 inches from the eye with near correction. *Each eye is covered separately and the small print (20/30) should be readable.* Vision should clear by frequent blinking which clears tear film. The tear film may only clear for a second due to abnormalities of blinking.
Do not bend to tie your shoes or strain in the bathroom.

Bruising of eyelid, facial, and even neck tissues
There is often redness in the skin that may involve the lower eyelid, cheek, and rarely the neck area especially if the lower eyelids underwent surgery. This gravitational effect may be evident from the upper eyelids to the lower lids one to two days after surgery as well. The tissue planes of the face allow dissection of blood induced by the surgical trauma to spread dependently by gravity from the upper eyelid into the lower eyelid, cheek, and even the neck. Remember the blood that accumulates from any bruise will turn color from red to blue, to brown, and finally to yellow as it is absorbed by the circulating blood capillaries and the lymphatic drainage systems of the face. Bruising should be distinguished from redness, pain, and swelling of the tissues due to infection. Infection rarely starts before three days after surgery.

Eyelid color changes as a bruise resolves are outlined below. The bruising pattern as outlined above occurs in the eyelid and gravitates to the lower face.

Bright red like---->dark red to maroon---->blue----->yellow and brown
a paint brush
Day 1–3   Day 3–5   Day 6–7   Day 8–9
                                                           after surgery

This same bruising process also affects the eyes. The eyes may be
swollen and there may be "jelly" bulging over eyelid lower eyelid margin
which is swollen conjunctiva (clear layer) which covers white sclera.
Subconjunctival space, a potential space between white sclera and the
normally clear conjunctiva, fills with fluid and may appear red due to
an admixture of blood.

Use of Ice for first four days
Ice should be used almost constantly (**the first 48 hours after surgery
except when sleeping**) to constrict the blood vessels, which decreases
the inflammatory response the body mounts in the eyelids and also
decreases the risks of bleeding into the eyelids. The head should be elevated as well. I recommend ice for 15 minutes every hour while awake
for the first 48 hours and then four times a day for an additional two
days.

Transient Double vision
Transient double vision (two images that do not clear with blinking)
should be noted and reported to the surgeon. Double vision should be
distinguished from blurred or fuzzy vision. Both double vision and
blurred vision may occur due to tearing or a drooping eyelid position
that partially obstructs the pupil. Rarely, double vision may result from
the local anesthetic injected at the time surgery. In this circumstance,
the extraocular muscles (muscles that move the eye) are temporarily
weakened for only a few hours after surgery. Double vision that persists
into the next day should be reported to your surgeon.

The best management of unfavorable results of eyelid surgery
Avoiding complications and carefully evaluation and treatment of any such complications promptly should they occur is of prime importance. Informed and educated patients tolerate unfavorable results with minimal stress if they have confidence in the surgeon and are prepared for the entire surgical experience as well as the possible complications that may arise after surgery. The purpose of this book is to prepare patients for such circumstances.

In general, when problems do occur after surgery, they can be overcome when the surgeon and patient work together. It is important for the surgeon to reassure patients who experience an unfavorable result and provide extra time and needed care to help any patient through the particular problem until its resolution. The cooperation of the patient is also crucial. Patients must contact their physicians with any change in their condition. A busy surgeon may have 5 to 10 postoperative patients per week and he can only provide the necessary help when he is contacted.

At times, referral to another specialist is important. The referral should be from the surgeon rather than upon the advice of a friend or another surgeon since the original surgeon knows the problem better than anyone else and that surgeon can provide appropriate information for any consultant. Fragmented, disjointed care results when patients seek many opinions.

The following compendium of unfavorable results and their management are provided.

Bleeding the first 48 hours after surgery
Should any bleeding occur, pressure is placed over the involved area for five minutes. The eyeball itself should not be directly pressed. The sterile

gauze should rest on the underlying bone surfaces. Firm pressure with the flat portion of the finger tips should be applied over the eye. After five minutes of direct pressure, bleeding should cease. If bleeding does not stop, reapply pressure for an additional five minutes. As soon as the bleeding stops, ice compresses should be applied over the involved eye. Patients should resume their antihypertensive medications immediately after surgery. High blood pressure may contribute to unnecessary bleeding. Check your blood pressure if you are use to doing so and call your physician even if the bleeding stops. Again, it is important to keep the head elevated and not to bend forward.

Tylenol or even Percocet (Tylenol with synthetic codeine) for more severe pain should be used for excessive pain. Medication of any type is rarely needed after the first 24 hours. Pain increases blood pressure. Again, aspirin, nonsteroidal anti-inflammatory agent, vitamin E, Gingko, garlic supplements, ginseng, and Persantine should be scrupulously avoided.

A small amount of blood may often be seen on the pillow upon awakening the morning after surgery. This bleeding is not a problem as long as there is no active bleeding while awake. The use of eye shields protects the eyelid tissues from inadvertent trauma while tossing and turning in bed. Ideally, sleep on one's back with the head elevated.

Again, should bleeding continue, notify your doctor.

Massive hemorrhage, Potential Threat to Vision

Some intermittent drops of blood and even overt bleeding from the wound is not significant and is expected, to some extent, the first 24 to 48 hours after surgery. Bloody tears are common the first 24 to 48 hours after surgery and are not a cause for alarm. Bleeding of any type should not be a constant dripping. Any such bleeding should necessitate 5 minutes of pressure with a sterile (4 by 4) gauze without pressing the eye itself as outlined above. Bleeding from deep, orbital structures or bleeding that starts in the eyelid tissues and dissects around the eye has the potential to cause permanent visual loss.

In order to prevent such an unusual event from progressing, the patient checks the vision in each eye by covering the opposite eye. Reading glasses depending on the patient's age and refractive error may be necessary. In any event the vision before surgery in each eye should be similar to the vision after surgery. Occasionally, tearing or mucous on the eyelashes will distort vision. A sterile gauze soaked in boiled water after it is cooled is applied to the eyelashes. Frequent blinking should improve the vision if only for a few seconds to ascertain that there is no vision problem.

Bleeding from the eyelid wound may create a serious problem. The blood may be confined within the unyielding bony orbit and around and behind the eye. Orbital hemorrhage will increase the pressure within the orbit and if the blood is trapped, result in external pressure on the eyeball and the optic nerve. Such pressure may compress the delicate blood supply to the eye and potentially cause irreversible optic nerve damage and visual loss.

Significant bleeding from the wound is accompanied by severe pain, double vision, or loss of vision. The eyelids become extremely tight and will not move.

Dr. Mauriello's Commentary: Severe hemorrhage is an extremely rare problem that demands emergency care by an expert ophthalmologist or ophthalmic plastic and reconstructive surgeon (orbital surgeon). This problem is avoided by a judicious surgeon who instructs his patients on proper medical care including elective control of blood pressure and avoidance of medications that cause bleeding. In addition, during surgery, patients with abnormal bleeding may be detected by the surgeon and appropriate treatment including aborting the cosmetic procedure is initiated.

Fortunately, this occurrence is extremely rare and has not been observed by the author in over 20 years of practice in over 15,000 procedures. I had occasion to treat a single patient who was undergoing eyelid reconstruction, not cosmetic surgery. This elderly gentleman developed an eyelid hemorrhage that necessitated delaying surgery. Such a hemorrhage may accompany any intraocular procedure such as cataract extraction and it is the standard of care to delay surgery in such rare instances.

Bleeding is most likely to occur within 48 hours of surgery and will be evident to the patient.

> *Dr. Mauriello's Commentary:* **If significant bleeding occurs as described above,** the patient should immediately contact their physician and go to the emergency room. A "911" call is appropriate to insure prompt transportation to the emergency room. Blood clotting tests are performed in the emergency room and blood pressure is monitored and controlled. Only an ophthalmologist and preferably an oculoplastic (orbital surgeon) are able to appropriately handle this problem.

Again, contact your doctor but proceed to the nearest emergency room for care. When you arrive in the emergency room, your physician will meet you. At the same time, the physician in charge of the emergency room will probably check blood pressure, blood count, and blood clotting (PT, PTT, platelet count, and bleeding time). It is important that your surgeon determine any prior tendency toward hemorrhage which may be re-evaluated along with your blood pressure in an emergency setting.

Medical treatment involves ice compresses and medications to lower the orbital pressure and blood pressure, if necessary. Emergency treatment under surgeon supervision involves elevation of the head, ice packs, topical medication to decrease the eye pressure, and oral medication to decrease fluid in the eye as well as the external pressure in the orbit.

Sometimes, the wounds are open to allow blood to escape from the eyelid and orbital tissues. Rarely, when the increased pressure on the optic nerve is so severe or if there is no response to medical treatment, emergency surgery is necessary to decompress the orbit by removing bone in the operating room.

Surgical treatment may be indicated. In such cases, the eyelid wounds may be surgically opened and any bleeding vessels cauterized. I have never had loss of vision due to hemorrhage or any permanent effects on any of my patients. As an oculoplastic consultant, I have personally encountered it many times on other patients due to a variety of causes. Rarely, hemorrhage occurs within the optic nerve sheath (detected by emergency CT scan of the orbit) that surrounds the optic nerve and the nerve substance is compressed by blood. In such cases, a window in the optic nerve sheath is surgically fashioned during emergency surgery. Prognosis may be related to the duration of the compression and by the severity of the hemorrhage.

Days Two to Five after Surgery
Tearing is often noted and should be combated by more frequent and complete blinking and topical artificial tears such as Refresh eye drops.

As stated above, all topical tears are over-the-counter. Burning, tearing, and even foreign body sensation occur due to incomplete blinking and consequent drying. Tylenol may relieve soreness that facilitates blinking which decreases drying and discomfort. Tears may be necessary every hour until the eye is sufficiently lubricated and comfortable. The frequency of the tears is then decreased to 2 hour intervals, then to every 3 hours, and finally 4 hour intervals.

In patients with mild exposure of the eyes due to incomplete blinking during the healing phase, forced blinking of the eyes and topical lubricants a few times a day usually controls symptoms until eyelid function returns over the next several days. As stated above, symptoms of dry eye include progressive itching, burning, foreign body sensation, pain, redness of the conjunctiva, corneal erosion, and even infection. If the eye is most irritated in the morning, lagophthalmos (incomplete closure of the eyelids) during sleep is a problem. A nonpreserved topical lubricating ointment such as Refresh PM or a gel-like drop (Refresh Celluvisc) will coat the eye if applied at bedtime (Refresh Liquigel, available in a bottle, is less viscous than Refresh Celluvisc and is sometimes more appealing to patients). Applying additional drops during the night upon awakening will improve the problem. Patients are encouraged to forcefully blink after surgery and also to massage the lower eyelid upward to lubricate the lower cornea that is most affected by incomplete excursion of the scarred upper eyelid.

Rarely, topical lubricants in the form of ointments as often as every hour are necessary. Ointments blur vision and may be alternated with drops to avoid constant blurred vision. In some patients, a punctal plug is necessary or even additional eyelid surgery (See Chapter 6 Postoperative Complications). Dry eye may also cause light sensitivity or photophobia. Dark glasses with side-panels or shields that keep light out of the eye and prevent wind from irritating the eyes are important adjunctive aids for comfort. Avoid direct blowing of air conditioners fans and heaters both within the car and at home from drying your eyes. Topical lubricants kept in the refrigerator are especially soothing. A foreign body sensation may be due to corneal irritation and requires a phone call to the physician should the discomfort not improve with topical tears.

Any inability to close the eye or **lagophthalmos** by a mm (1/25th) is noted by the surgeon. Lagophthalmos is more likely to occur when sleeping since only gentle closure is possible and is usually transient. Forced closure of the eyelids is not present during sleep. A family member may detect subtle inability to close the eye while the patient is sleeping. A flashlight may be necessary as in the patient photographed below. The patient is encouraged to look down and blink slowly to moisten the lower one-third of the cornea.

Each surgery performed on the delicate eyelid inevitably causes irreversible scarring and may reduce the casual blink, forced voluntary closure of the eyelids, and result in lagophthalmos (inability to close the eye).

Overall less swelling, less pain, and less mucous are present after each advancing day after surgery. If increased pain, tightness, or mucous are present, suspect infection. You should call your doctor. Infection is treated with oral antibiotics. As stated above, itching suggests topical allergy to ophthalmic drops which should be discontinued and your physician notified. Itching or allergy may start the day of surgery while infection usually starts in 3 to 5 days after surgery.

DAY 3 AFTER SURGERY Bruising of the upper and lower eyelids is evident. Steri-strips support the lower eyelid while it is swollen and healing and help to maintain the cheek in slightly upward position. This patient had underlying dry eye and required topical tears for mild irritation for approximately 3 weeks.

One week after Surgery
The redness and swelling significantly dissipate. With time, the redness turns blue, then brown and finally yellow as the blood products in the contused areas are broken down physiologically. Warm compresses should be used as long as bruising is present and swelling persists. These compresses promote healing by increasing the blood supply to the injured area. Swelling or edema is always worse in the morning and improves during the day due to movement of fluid by gravity from the eyelids to the lower face as the patient assumes an erect position. Sleeping with extra pillows keeps the head elevated and reduces eyelid swelling. If possible, the patient should sleep on his (her) back to avoid inadvertent trauma to the area.

Day 7 after Surgery (above)—eyelid swelling has markedly decreased and bruising is now more brownish yellow in color than red.

Numbness of the eyelid skin and Use of Eye Make-up After Surgery
Makeup may be used after 10 to 14 days after consulting your surgeon. On occasion, patients note numbness of the eyelids when applying makeup. This numbness is transitory but may rarely persist 6 months to a year after surgery. The nerves that supply the eyelids are just beneath the orbicularis muscle. The orbicularis oculi muscle is just beneath the thin eyelid skin. Such sensory nerves are rarely injured and sometimes take several weeks to months to regenerate. A patient has never complained to me of permanent numbness of the overlying eyelid or facial skin after cosmetic eyelid surgery.

Long-term Surgical Outcomes

In 95 to 98% of surgeries in my experience, you will usually be quite happy with the result 4 weeks after surgery. Eyelid swelling generally takes 3 months to resolve but it may be persistent for one year. I have seen a case where conjunctival edema (jelly) persisted and required additional surgery. It is virtually impossible to remove all excess skin and fat without causing complications (inability to close the eye or lower eyelid paladin) or "an operated" look. Surgeons strive to produce a natural appearance to the eyelid anatomy so that patients look refreshed. The eyelid shape should ideally not change. The surgery is restorative and, in Dr. Mauriello's opinion, should not create a new image or look. Patients may notice tightness of the eyelid skin for several months and rarely up to one year or longer after surgery. Rarely, if ever, does the entire eyelid surgery ever need to be repeated. At times, it is necessary to perform a touchup for a residual problem that was not fully corrected at the time of surgery. Any such touchup should be delayed for a minimum of sixth months after surgery unless there is a functional risk to vision.

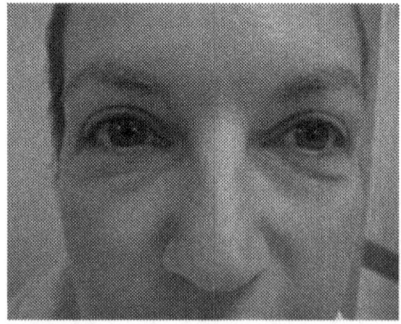

Figure 4
BEFORE

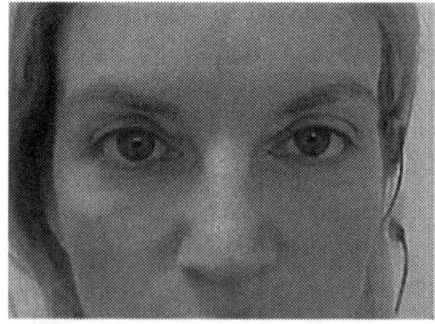

Figure 5
6 MONTHS AFTER SURGERY

Preoperative view (above left) and post-operative view (above right) show defined upper eyelid creases and platform between the upper eyelid lashes and the eyelid crease. The lower eyelids appear less baggy after surgery and the upper cheek is elevated after surgery.

> **Dr. Mauriello's commentary:** *Note cheek elevation after surgery. Patient indicated that her appearance gradually continued to improve up to six months after surgery.*

Undercorrection always better than overcorrection

It is always preferable to undercorrect than to perform too much surgery. It is far easier to remove additional tissues than to replace eyelid skin or fat that was removed excessively. Excision of too much skin in the upper eyelid may inhibit eyelid closure and in very unusual circumstances require skin grafting to restore normal eyelid function. Excision of too much skin in the lower eyelid may result in lower eyelid pull down and may exacerbate a pre-existing dry eye due to exposure of the eyeball. This condition generally improves and, in many cases, resolves with massage. Rarely, the corner of the eye needs to be resuspended to tighten the lower eyelid. Your surgeon often prevents this complication at the time of the blepharoplasty since lower eyelid laxity is noted at the time of the office consultation and surgically repaired at the time blepharoplasty is performed.

Even more rarely, a skin grafting procedure is necessary to elevate the lower eyelid. I have never had to place a skin graft for any of my patients or re-suspend a lateral (outer corner of the eye) canthus after cosmetic surgery.

Section 5

SKIN CARE

CHAPTER 7

How Do I take care of my skin before and after eyelid surgery? Botox® and Restylane ® treatment after cosmetic eyelid surgery

Importance of Skin Care

Skin care helps to protect the skin against photoaging (aging due to sun exposure) and skin cancer. Skin care products improve uneven pigmentation and possibly thicken the skin. Ultimately, skin care enhances the beneficial effects of eyelid surgery. This section considers over-the-counter as well as prescription medications. A background discussion above the anatomy of the skin is helpful.

> *Dr. Mauriello's commentary: It is important to maintain the effect of the surgery.* Ask your surgeon about skin care. Such care is also important to help prevent skin cancers.

Anatomy of the skin

The skin consists of a superficial epidermis and an underlying dermis. The subcutaneous tissue is beneath the dermis.

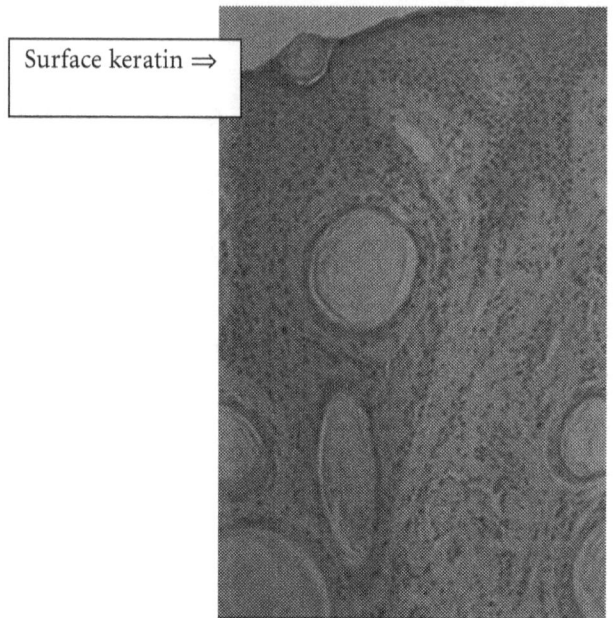

Surface keratin ⇒

Figure 1
MICROSCOPIC SECTION OF SKIN WITH
HAIR FOLLICLE
(CIRCULAR STRUCTURES).

The dermis has two layers: a superficial papillary layer with rich network of capillaries and deeper and thicker reticular (net-like structure) layer. The papillary layer is so termed because it has connective tissue whose role is supportive. The papillary layer has papillae (ridges) which project into the adjacent overlying epidermis. The rich capillary plexus (network) lies within each papilla and nourishes the overlying epidermis. The papillary dermis also has small veins or venules that form a flat bed below the bases of the papillae and is composed of connective tissue that is less compact than the reticular dermis. Eyelid skin has a flat dermal epidermal junction with few and less developed ridges or papillae but a thinner and denser dermis.

The outermost layer of skin or epidermis is composed of epithelial cells which have a protective role. The most superficial part of the epidermis is the stratum corneum or horny layer which is produced by the epidermis and composed of keratin. The keratin in the straum corneum protects against physical damage but also, to some extent, against sun exposure. It is most developed on the palms of the hands and the soles of the feet.

Melanin, the brown skin pigment, is present in the epidermis and like melanin throughout the body is produced by specialized cells known as melanocytes. The melanin protects the skin surface against ultraviolet light by absorbing it. For this reason, skin cancers do not occur in blacks.

Hair follicles are associated with sebaceous glands that express their sebum or oily into the lumen of the hair follicle to serve as an inherent cool cream for the lubrication of the overlying skin. The great number of pilosebaceous units distinguish facial from skin outside the face. The nose and forehead have more sebaceous units than the cheeks or temples.

With age, the hairs turn gray due to decreased production of melanin by melanocytes in the bulbs of the hair follicle. At the eyelid margin, there are no pillar (hairs) units associated with sebaceous units. This isolated sebaceous unit, unassociated with a hair follicle, is also unique to the papillae of breasts, labia minora (of the vagina), and corners of the lips against to vermillion border. In the soles of the feet and palms of the hands, there are no sebaceous glands or hair follicles.

The sweat gland has a secretory part (part of the gland that secretes the substance produced by the gland). The secretory portion is in the sub-cutaneous tissue below the papillary and reticular dermis. The duct (conduit or passageway for the secretion from the gland) of the sweat gland is a small tube that allows secretion onto the skin surface. It courses through the dermis to the skin surface. Along with the complex blood supply to the skin whose flow to skin is influenced by external as well as internal temperature changes, sweat helps to regulate body temperature.

When laser resurfacing wounds extend below the mid reticular dermis, that is, to the level of the deep reticular dermis, irreversible scar tissue formation may result.

LAYERS OF SKIN:

epidermis
papillary dermis
reticular dermis
subcutaneous tissue

FULL THICKNESS EYELID

Skin side of eyelid

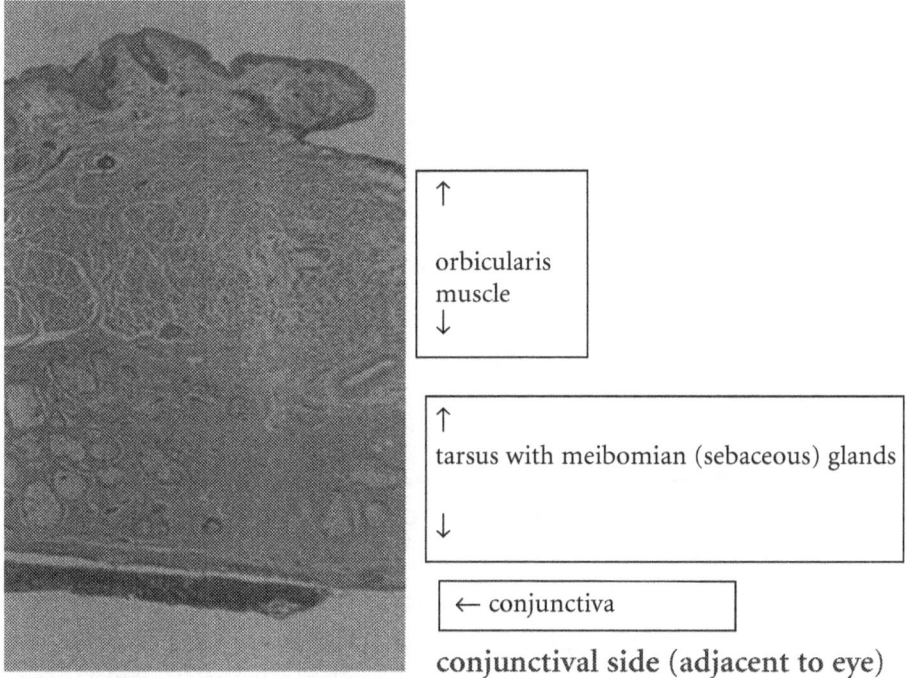

orbicularis
muscle

tarsus with meibomian (sebaceous) glands

← conjunctiva

conjunctival side (adjacent to eye)

Figure 2

The eyelid skin is extremely skin and bundles of orbicularis muscle lie just beneath it. The tarsus is a fibrous structure is the backbone of the eyelids and it contains sebaceous glands that produce the oily tear film layer. The epithelium of the tarsus is the conjunctiva and since it is a mucosal surface it does not contain keratin.

The conjunctiva has no hair follicles associated with sebaceous glands or sweat glands.

PHOTOAGING (AGING DUE TO SUN EXPOSURE)

So-called **photoaging** of the skin results from ultraviolet (UV) light exposure and is cumulative over years. Sun damage results in the following changes in the skin:

o   wrinkles, dark blotches

o   freckles, leathery texture

o   loss of elasticity.

In addition, the skin is predisposed to skin cancers such as basal cell carcinoma, squamous cell carcinoma, and melanoma. Sun blocks are absolutely essential in preventing these cancers and should be used by everyone.

HISTOLOGY of Photoaging or sun damaged skin

With age and sun damage, the superficial epidermis of the skin gradually losses its translucency and appears dry, rough, and dull skin, and so-called benign keratosis develop. In addition, ephelides (freckles) are noted in increased numbers due to accumulation of granules of the brown pigment (melanin) in the lower layer of cells of the epidermis, known as the basal and suprabasal keratinocytes. The keratinocytes are the cells that constitute the epidermis.

In addition, the normal elastic tissue in the dermis of the skin breaks down. Macrophages are specialized cells that repair damage and degeneration throughout the tissues of the body by engulfing the broken down coarse granules. The elastotic breakdown material accumulates and crowds out the normal collagenous fibers which are also degenerating and resorbing with age. The normal collagen fibers provide the framework of the skin. The elastotic material is resorbed and ultimately the total volume of the dermis diminishes. Since there is relatively too much epidermis for the shrinking dermis, wrinkles appear on the skin surface.

There is also loss of hyaluronic acid that makes up the ground substance or milieu that contains the collagen fibers. The ground substance or matrix of the dermis contains glycosaminoglycans (GAG's) such as hyaluronic acid that attracts water and thereby provides hydration for the skin. Tissue levels of hyaluronic acid decrease with age and add to the shrinkage of the dermis.

> *Restylane ® is a stable form of hyaluronic acid, so-called molecularly bound form, that when injected into wrinkles attracts water, restores volume, and reduces wrinkles by plumping up the tissues.* **Its effects last 6 months or longer.**

The melanocyte is a specialized cell that produces the skin pigment, melanin. Melanocytes increase in number in the lower or basal layer of epidermis and result in solar lentigos (liver spot) in which the amount of melanin or brown pigment increases in each melanocyte and also in the basal keratinocytes (cells of the epidermis at its lowest portion). Specialized macrophages, known as dermal melanophages, migrate into the dermis with the sole purpose of imbibing and digesting dispersed melanin pigment). In addition, comedones that plug the openings of pilosebaceous units develop with photoaging or sun damage.

SUN BLOCK

An effective sun block is the basis of all skin care. Excess ultraviolet B (UV.) rays occur in 290-320nm cause skin burns while UVAII short rays (320-340nm) and UVAI long rays (340-400nm) are responsible for photoaging. *These latter rays may lead to skin cancer.*

Zine oxide is a sun block. A sun block creates a *physical* block to the sun rays. A sun block is not absorbed by the body and provides broad spectrum protection against UVA/UVB. from 290 nm to 380 nm.

SUN SCREEN

In contrast to a sun block, a sun screen is absorbed by the superficial epidermis and metabolized or broken down by the body to potentially cause allergy.

The most common chemical sun screen, octyl methoxycinnamate (OMC), is absorbed by the epidermis of the skin. It only blocks the UVB. burning rays, not the long UVA rays that cause photoaging. Other sun screens have similarly narrow zones of protection.

In summary, sun blocks are superior to sun screens since they inhibit the damaging effects of broad spectrum of ultraviolet light. In addition, the sun block is not absorbed by the epidermis of the skin and, therefore, allergy is much less likely to develop.

ANTIOXIDANTS

In addition to sun screens and sun blocks, antioxidants protect against photoaging by neutralizing reactive oxygen species or free radicals which damage skin at the cellular level. A free radical is an atom or group of atoms with at least one unpaired election. Each unpaired electron looks for another electron with which to bond and chemical reactions occur until each unpaired electron has a mate. Sun (UV) exposure, smoking, and pollution deplete antioxidants.

Antioxidants—Vitamin C and E, zinc, alpha lipoic acid, and dihy-drolipolate, glutathione

Topical vitamin-C (L-Ascorbic acid form) is a powerful antioxidant that in the laboratory enhances collagen (fibrous tissue formation) synthesis. Vitamin C products, in general, improve skin tone, elasticity and firmness of skin by collagen synthesis and prevent photoaging by their antioxidant effect. Aging skin as previously discussed is characterized by loss of collagen. The ability of collagen to actually thicken the skin is not substantiated by my personal observation.

Vitamin C derivatives such as ascorbyl palmitate and magnesium ascorbyl phosphate, commonly found in many skin care products, are not absorbed or converted to the active L-ascorbic acid form in high enough concentrations to have an antioxidant effect. It is important that vitamin C is pure, bioavailable (the active vitamin C penetrates the skin) and stable. Concentrations for the eyelids are lower (5%) than in the facial area (10–20%) in order to avoid skin irritation and redness. The eyelid creams or gels smooth the puffy appearance of eyelids.

Vitamin E is dependent on vitamin C because it helps regenerate vitamin E. Both vitamin C and E prevent suppression of immunity induced by sun exposure (UV light), have anti-inflammatory effects, and promote healing. Alpha lipoic acid regenerates vitamin C. Only vitamin E or alpha tocopheral is the stable, active form. Vitamin E esters (acetate, succinate linoleate, nicotinate) found in many cosmetic foundations are not antioxidants.

Zinc works similarly to vitamin C but does not help regenerate vitamin. E. However, zinc helps the body maintain proper levels blood levels of Vitamin. E. Zinc stabilizes lipid or cell membranes. Zinc and bioflavonoids tend to firm and smooth skin.

Products that high concentrations of antioxidants, are stable, and have superior bioavailabilty. Skin creams have more of a moisturizing effect than creams.

RETINOIDS OR TRETINOINS (RETIN-A)

Retinoids are a great advance in skin care and these require a physician's prescription. Their effects are quite dramatic when they are used assiduously and judiciously as prescribed by your surgeon or dermatologist.

Retin-A (Ortho Pharmaceutical Corporation, Raritan, NJ) has the following well demonstrated effects:

- helps decrease hyperpigmentation (dark pigmentation) and, therefore, may be helpful after laser resurfacing or chemical peel
- increases collagen formation (new fibrous tissue formation)
- promotes healing which is useful after any injury including chemical peels, laser resurfacing, and dermabrasion
- promotes new blood vessel formation associated with healing (angiogenesis) which may lead to prolonged skin erythema (redness)

Tretinoin has the following effects on the skin at the cellular level that are responsible for the above effects:
- decreases the thickness of stratum corneum (horny outer layer of the skin's superficial epidermal layer)
- exfoliates retained keratin (superficial horny outer protective layer of the epidermis of skin) from hair follicles

- decreases dysplasia and atypia (premalignant changes) of the normal superficial epidermal maturation

- decreases epidermal melanin (brown skin pigment) and thereby promotes uniform dispersion of melanin granules

- depletes dermal melanophages (specialized macrophages that engulf melanin pigment) and cause pigmentary changes in the skin (dyschromia)

- increases collagen gene expression in fibroblast cultures

- reconstitutes papillary dermis (superficial supportive layer of dermis)

- increases dermal collagen synthesis

- increases new blood vessels (angiogenesis)

Renova (Ortho Pharmacetualical Corporation) contains tretinoin 0.05% in a water case. It may diminish irritant dermatosis that may occur with Retin-A.

Tretinoins cause skin redness and flakiness
The main problem with retinoins is the irritation they induce. Redness (erythema), flakiness, and increased skin sensitivity persist 2–4 weeks after treatment. This irritation often subsides if treatment is continued. There may be a true allergy to butylated hydroxytoluene, a perservative used. In this case, the product needs to be discontinued.

Use tretinoins at night
A light sensitivity (photosensitivity) may result from thinning of the stratum corneum. Sunlight may breakdown tretinoin and, therefore, tretinoin should be used at night. Tretinoin induced photosensitivity may be exacerbated by thiazides, tetracyclines, phenothiazines, fluroquinolones and sulfonamides.

The preparation should be chosen which is least irritating and should start with lowest concentration. Tretinoin is available as follows (the cream is more moisturizing):

Retin-A cream	0.025
	0.05%
	0.1%
Retin-A gel	0.01%
	0.025%
Retin-A solution	0.05%
Renova (water in light mineral oil emulsion)	0.05%
Retina-A Microcream	0.1%

Renova and Retin-A Microcream may be less irritating. The latter forms microscopic porous beads without the use of oils or organize solvents like ethanol or acetone that may cause skin drying and irritation. A third generation tretinoin, adapalene (Differin) 0.1% gel (Galderma, Fort Worth, Texas), possibly produces less irritation and no phototoxicity. In addition, tretinoins may aggravate acne rosacea and atopic dermatitis as well as acne vulgaris (common acne).

Tretitoins should be applied to a clean well dried face at night. They should be started on an every other night basis and gradually increased to nightly use. In patients with sensitive skin and during the summer, tretinoins may be started every third night. All abrasive soaps, cleansers, and scrubs should be discontinued. Any high concentration of alcohol and astringents with their drying effect should be scrupulously avoided. Wait 30 minutes before applying a moisturizer after tretinoin.

Tazarotene is a retinoid that is helpful in the treatment of psoriasis, acne vulgaris, and photoaging. Clinical studies have shown that tazarotene 0.1% gel has greater activity against acne vulgaries than tretinoin (Retin-A 0.025% gel, Retin-A Micro 0.1%) and adapalene (Differin) 0.1% gel. Adverse events consist primarily of irritation, peeling, erythema, dryness, burning, and itching. They are most common during the first 1–2 weeks of therapy and can be minimized with use of the cream formulation, alternate day application, short contact therapy, mild cleansers, and combination therapy.

OTHER OVER-THE-COUNTER SKIN CARE PRODUCTS
In addition to sun blocks and screens, and the tretinoins, other products are helpful and the consumer should be knowledgeable about.

Aloe, rosemary, cucumber, and green tea are calming botanical extracts which also have anti-inflammatory effects and help soothe, lightens, and refresh tired, sagging skin. **Chamomile** has a soothing and calming, emollient or soothing and softening effect. **Thyme extract** helps to soothe skin by increasing blood circulation and combined with thyme extract help soften but not eliminate the dark circles under the eye. There are no controlled studies to demonstrate the efficacy of these products although many such products are touted commercially.

In contrast, **alpha hydroxy acids (glycolic and lactic acid)** have a long track record of exfoliating the rough, textured outer layer of skin and thereby smoothing the skin.

Other common alpha-hydroxy carbolic acids—
> mandolin acid
> malic acid
> tartaric acid
> citric acid
> pyruvic acid
> benzylic acid
> tropic acid

kojic acid lightens skin by inhibiting production of melanin

Alpha-hydroxy acids (AHAs)—thicken epidermis, collagen in papillary dermis, and ground substance in dermis
AHA's help to thicken the skin by thickening the epidermis and the papillary dermis (superficial dermis) with new collagen and acid mucopolysaccharide, the material in dermis' ground substance. The quality of elastic fibers improves as does the even distribution of brown melanin. AHA's also cause diminished abnormal keratinization. There may be less irritation than with tretinoins.

Combining AHA's with tretinoins may not cause any greater irritation than with tretinoins alone and may improve dyspigmentation or abnormal skin pigmentation than with the use of tretinoin alone. Glycolic acids range from 40 to 70% and may be applied at weekly or biweekly time. The higher concentrations are used by your surgeons as chemical peels. AHA's tend to dry the skin but they may be used in the morning to a clean face.

Hydroquinones—prevents new melanin (brown pigment) formation
Hydroquinone does not bleach out existing pigment but does prevent the production of new brown melanin pigment in the skin. This drug inhibits tryosinase which is necessary for melanocytes in the skin to

continue to produce melanin, the brown skin pigment. Pigment irregularities with no visible changes in the skin usually result from sun exposure and are exacerbated by pregnancy and oral contraceptive use.

Irritation may result and the concentration from 3 to 4% up to 8% may be decreased. A solution or gel may be more irritating than a moisturizing cream base. In some patients, a hydrocortisone to decrease inflammation may be necessary.

> **WARNING: Patients with an unusual condition known as ochronosis may develop permanent brown discoloration within the dermis.**

The solution gel, or cream formation is used in the morning or twice daily. It may be combined as a 4 to 8% solution with retinoic acid 0.025% or 0.05% along with a corticosteroid (hydrocortisone 1–2.5% or triamcinolone 0.025% twice daily). These preparations should be combined with a suncreen or sunblock.

Melanex	*3% solution*		
Eloquin Forte	*4% cream*		
Solaquin Forte	*4% cream*	*with sunscreen*	*(Padimate O, Dioxybenzone, oxybenzone)*
Solaquin Forte	*4% get*	*with sunscreen*	*(Padimate O, oxybenzone)*
Eldopaque Forte	*4% cream*	*with tinted sunscreen*	*(iron oxides)*
Viquin Forte	*4% cream*	*with sunscreen*	*(Padimate O, Dioxybenzone, oxybenzone)*
Melquin-3	*3% solution*		
Melquin HP	*4% cream*		
Nuquin HP	*4% cream*	*with sunscreen*	*(Octyl methoxycinnamate, benzophenone)*

Nuquin HP   4% gel   with sunscreen (dioxybenzone)
Melpagque HP   4% cream   with tinted sunblock (iron oxides)

Kojic acid, another tyrosinase inhibitor, prevents formation of new melanin pigment. It is an extract from the fungus *Aspergillus aryzeau*. It may occasionally irritate the skin. Azelez (Allergan Pharmceuticals Inc. Irvine, CA) contains 20% azelaic acid and may be helpful for some patients.

Topical corticosteroids will increase angiogenesis (new blood formation) that is a disadvantage after laser resurfacing.

If there is a problem with tolerance to a hydroquinone prior to laser skin resurfacing, it is reasonable to discontinue the hydroquinone and treat hyperpigmentation should it arise after resurfacing.

TIMING OF APPLICATION OF SKIN TREAMENTS

Vitamin C products should be applied to a clean, well dried face in the morning. The sunblock is followed by make-up. Tretinoins should be applied to a clean well dried face at bedtime. Hydroquinone may be used in the morning. It is best to introduce only one treatment regimen at a time to decrease irritation or allergy. One must decide on the priorities of their treatment choices with their physician.

Laser Skin Resurfacing, Chemical Peel, Dermabrasion
The aging face has the following processes that cause sagging of skin and depressions in the face. Specifically, there is decreased skin thickness and elasticity. There is also gradual absorption of subcutaneous tissue and loosening of the firm attachments of the skin to the underlying layers. For example, these changes result in the gravitational descent of

soft tissues that accentuate the nasolabial groove, a line that extends from each side of the nose to the corners of the mouth (Friedland JA, Simultaneous laser resurfacing with face lift: A safe alternative for facial rejuvenation. *Aesthetic Surgery Journal.* 19:499, 1999). Static wrinkles should be distinguished from dynamic wrinkles. Dynamic wrinkles change with movement of the muscles underlying the skin of face that cause facial expression. Such dynamic wrinkles of the overlying skin change in response to contraction of the muscles of facial expression. The wrinkles or rhytides whether dynamic or static are virtual linear valleys within the skin due to loss of the collagen which is replaced by degenerating so-called elastic tissue. Rhytides are caused by such changes in the skin layer, the dermis, below the epidermis.

Blephapharoplasty and skin treatments including laser resurfacing, chemical peel, and dermabrasion are more effective in removing static wrinkles and have little, if any, effect on dynamic wrinkles.

The popularity of carbon dioxide and erbium laser skin resurfacing has waned in recent years. There are a host of new lasers introduced at a rapid rate. None to date have been demonstrated to produce results than are better than simple chemical peels.

Intense pulsed light treatments are effective in decreasing vascular red pigment on the skin surface and brown age spots but less effective in reducing wrinkles.

In addition to chemical peels, mechanical dermabrasion is helpful in treating raised scars. The results may be less predictable and measured than with the laser where the energy delivered to the tissues is specifically measured. The effect of the peel is dependent on the exact solution and its concentration, the length of time it contacts the skin, and the skin type and thickness. The greatest long-term complication of all these techniques is permanent lack of pigmentation and scarring. The neck area is particularly prone to scarring because of its lack of hair follicles. The hair follicles provide the epithelium which relines the treated skin.

INITIAL SKIN TREATMENT FOR PIGMENTARY (Irregular skin blotching) SKIN CHANGES PRIOR TO SKIN REJUVENATION (Chemical peels or laser skin resurfacing)
Minimizing sun exposure and the use of sunscreens is necessary at all times. Retinoic acid 0.1% and 4% hydroquinone for 6 weeks are helpful in patients with minimal skin damage due to sun exposure. Only a few patients with minimal pigment changes respond to this simple and nonaggressive treatment. (Baker TM Chemicals and lasers for skin resurfacing. *Aesthetic Surgery Journal* 1999; 19:325-327). Hydroquinone may not be necessary since the rejuvenating chemical peel or laser resurfacing destroys all pigment and hydroquinone only prevents new pigmentation.

Alpha hydroxy acids or glycolic acid 30% to 70% are used over several visits in progressively increasing concentrations to abrade the superficial epidermis which has pigment bearing cells (melanocytes) at the basal or lower level of the epidermis. These treatments are suited for younger working woman who have only superficial skin changes and neither require nor have the time for more involved procedures.

If patients with pigmentary changes are not improved sufficiently with the above regimen (glycolic acid or hydroquinone), then a trichloroacetic acid (TCA) peel may be helpful. A 35% TCA full face peel is accompanied in the office without any anesthetic and heals generally in 5–10 days. Redness of the skin lasts 2 to 3 weeks. Superficial lines improve.

Dr. Mauriello's patients have used Physicians choice of Arizona Products since 2000. These products are only available to licensed physicians and aestheticians. Home care regimens individualized by skin type are complemented by self-neutralizing peels performed by Dr. Mauriello in the office. These peels enhance home care regimens. Various types of peels are provided, but all are self-neutralizing with minimal redness, flaking, and downtime. Dr. Mauriello's patients have found that the home care maintence and office peels improve the quality of the skin and enhance the effect of cosmetic eyelid surgery.

Botox® and Restylane ® treatment after cosmetic eyelid surgery
Both Botox® and Restylane ® described below complement the effects of cosmetic eyelid surgery. Botox improves wrinkles without the permanent effects of surgery. The results may be cumulative.

> *Dr. Mauriello's Commentary: The office procedure is done over the lunch hour and after treatment, the patient is able to drive home. Botox is best for the upper face (forehead lines, nasal lines, and crow's feet in the corners of the eye). It may be used to enhance the mouth and lips as well especially when complemented by Restylane®. Dr. Mauriello pioneered the use of Botox and was one of the first physicians in the New York metropolitan area to incorporate Botox into his practice in 1983 to treat eyelid spasms.*

Restylane is a naturally occurring substance and its effects last probably twice as long as collagen treatments. Skin testing is necessary with collagen but not with Restylane®. The Restylane effect is prolonged since local muscle contractions weakened by Botox® do not spread the Restylane® and dissipate its effects. When Botox® and Restylane® are combined with eyelid surgery, the entire face may be further improved.

Some background on both of these substances is provided for the readers.

History of Botox®

Allergan's BOTOX® product was approved by the FDA for clinical use in 1989, and has a proven track record for the treatment of strabismus (crossed eyes) and blepharospasm (involuntary eyelid spasms). In December, 2000, Botox® was also approved for the treatment of abnormal head position and neck pain associated with cervical dystonia. Botox® Cosmetic was approved for the treatment of glabellar (between the eyebrows) frown and scowl lines in Canada in April, 2001 and in the United States in April, 2002.

Medical Uses of Botox

As of 2000, BOTOX® therapy is approved in 70 countries for a broad range of medical conditions and is currently being investigated in the U.S. for the treatment of:

- hyperhidrosis (excessive sweating)
- post-stroke muscle spasticity
- juvenile cerebral palsy
- spasticity including back spasm
- pain and headache including myofascial pain
- management of occupational dystonia (involuntary movement)
- writer's cramp
- temporomandibular disorders
- gastrointestinal disease
- urologic disorders
- tremors

- tics

- cosmetic uses

How does Botox® work?

Botox blocks the nerve impulses that cause a voluntary skeletal muscle to contract. Botox ® is, therefore, called a "neurotoxin." Botox ® binds to special sites at terminals where the nerve and muscle interface. These terminals are known as motor nerve terminals. Specifically, Botox ® blocks the release of a chemical that causes the muscle to contract. This chemical is called "acetylcholine" and is known as a neurotransmitter, Actually, Botox, the neurotoxin, cleaves to a special protein, the so-called "SNAP-25 protein" that is necessary for the release of the acetylcholine. Without the release of the acetylcholine, the muscle affected by the particular nerve terminal is unable to contract. Botox does not inactivate every tiny muscle fiber and, therefore, does not generally lead to complete loss of muscle function. The effect of Botox is temporary and eventually after 3 to 6 months, muscle contraction return. At that time, the wrinkle becomes evident but usually after successive treatments, the wrinkle never becomes as noticeable as when it was first treated.

What is Botox ® Cosmetic?

Botox® Cosmetic (Botulinum Toxin Type A) is a purified Neurotoxin Complex. It is a sterile vacuum-dried purified botulinum toxin type A, produced from a strain of bacterium, *Clostridium botulinum* type A. The bacterium is grown in a specific culture. The culture is then purified and the resulting complex is dissolved in a sterile sodium chloride solution that contains human albumin and is sterile filtered. The drug is received in the physician's office in its frozen state in a vial.

Is Botox a poison?

Botox is the same chemical that causes botulism. This condition causes death by weakening the muscles of respiration. The drug is a toxin in sufficiently high doses but is extremely safe in the dosages used to treat wrinkles. Any drug is potentially a poison if given in sufficient dose. Botulinum toxin was only known for its toxic effects until its therapeutic effects were appreciated and developed by Dr. Alan Scott, an ophthalmologist at Pacific Medical Center in the late 1970's. He developed the drug to treat crossed eyes in children and adults. Every drug has an LD-50. The LD-50 is the dose of a drug that given in an experimental system will cause 50% of mice injected with a given dose to die.

> *Dr. Mauriello's Commentary: It is estimated that 40 vials of Botox, each of which contains 100 units, are toxic to humans. Generally, one-quarter to one-half of a vial is injected in the facial regions for cosmetic indications.*

The injections of Botox in the desired doses represent extremely small quantities of the drug and the only way Botox will cause a problem is if the injection is given in a muscle that has a critical function or an inadvertent overdose is given. In order to have continued therapeutic effect, Botox needs to be re-injected at certain intervals because its effect wears off at the site it is injected.

Does the drug affect my whole body?
The drug is injected at the site where its effects are desired. Minute amounts are not detectable in the blood when given in doses in the therapeutic range. Nonetheless, when sensitive studies called single fiber electromyography are performed to measure minute muscle activity, the effects of the drug are measurable at sites distant from the injection.

Are there potential unreported or unknown side-effects?
There is always the extremely rare risk of an unknown side-effect with any drug. The drug has been FDA approved for other uses since 1988.

Dr. Mauriello has treated several hundred patients with this drug since 1983. Some patients have received as many 30 injections over the years since the effects are temporary and repeat injections are necessary. As a result, he has personally given over 6000 injections and has noted only minimal side effects.

What are some of the more common, possible side-effects?
The possible side effects are listed below.

Pain at injection site: The most common side-effect is mild pain on injection which dissipates almost immediately after the injection is given. There in no pain after the procedure and no medication is required.

Mild Bruising: There may be slight bruising at the site or even a small hematoma or collection of blood under the skin with minimal discomfort. As with any bruise, this problem resolves itself over 7 to14 days and may be treated, if desired, with ice the first 48 hours four times a day for 5 minutes (ice may be placed in a Ziploc bag). Make-up may be used to conceal any discoloration.

Headache, respiratory infection, Flu syndrome, and nausea: In clinical trials conducted by Allergan, Inc., the most frequently reported adverse events were studied. In this study, patients received either Botox or a placebo (a pseudo-drug without any pharmacologic effect). Patients reported the following side-effects without knowledge of what they had taken (the investigators had no knowledge as well):

	Botox Treated Group	Placebo (nontreated group)
Headache	13.3%	17.7%
Respiratory infection	3.5%	3.8%
Temporary eyelid droop	3.2%	0%
Nausea	3.0%	2.3%
Flu syndrome	2.0%	1.5%

Note that the incidence of all side-effects, except for the temporary eyelid droop, occurred significantly in the placebo group as well as the Botox group.

In Dr. Mauriello's experience, even the "most common" side-effects are extremely rare.

Ptosis (drooping) of the Upper Lid: Ptosis of the upper lid is rare. In treating facial lines in the forehead, your physician will selectively weaken the muscles that close the eyes. These latter muscles are anatomically close to the muscles that elevate the lid, and the potential to weaken the eyelid elevators exists.

Dr. Mauriello's comments regarding ptosis (drooping of the upper lid) after Botox injections: Dr. Mauriello has observed two cases of ptosis after several hundred Botox injections for cosmetic reasons. He examined a patient who was referred to him by a plastic surgeon. This patient developed ptosis subsequent to treatment elsewhere. Like virtually all side-effects, the ptosis subsequently resolved. The second patient had a pre-existing drooping lid. The technique of injection should virtually eliminate this rare, transient complication of Botox ®.

BOTOX® COSMETIC should not be used in the presence of infection at the proposed injection site(s).

Botox Allergy: As with any drug, serious allergic reaction may occur that necessitates treatment. Dr. Mauriello has encountered two patients with allergic reactions. Should a rash develop, your physician should be called. However, should a full-blown allergy (known as an anaphylactic reaction) including tightness of the throat and shortness of breath develop, emergency treatment at a hospital emergency room is warranted.

Dr. Mauriello has encountered only two patients with allergic reactions to Botox. Both patients experienced reactions to the experimental form of Botulinum toxin, type A, before it was approved by the FDA. One developed a skin rash when injected at two separate times, and the other developed a skin rash and a tightness of the throat. In both instances, the drug was no longer given.

Avoid Botox in pregnancy: Botox should not be used during pregnancy, since no testing has established its safety during pregnancy.

Muscle weakness: Systemic weakness or muscle paralysis may occur. Difficulty swallowing has occurred rarely after treatment of the neck muscles. The treatment of the neck should not usually exceed more than 30 units at one time.

Possible Drug Interactions: Botox should be used extremely judiciously in conjunction with certain drugs that interfere with neuromuscular activity. The drugs include antibiotics such as **amino-glycosides, curare, lincosamides, polymyxin antibiotics, quinidine, magnesium sulfate, anticholinesterases, and succinylcholine.** The physician who treats you will obtain a complete medical history that includes the history of medications you are talking. Always check with your physician if you have any concerns. In this regard, the drug should be used cautiously in any patient with a neuromuscular disease, including rare diseases such as myasthenia gravis.

None of the patients in Dr. Mauriello's practice has experienced a drug interaction.

Other possible Side-effects: Since Botox is produced and contains human albumin, there is an extremely remote risk of viral disease transmission. This risk is minimized by donor screening and the manufacturing processes. No documented case of Creutzfeld Jakob ("Mad Cow Disease") disease has been reported to date.

Antidote for overdose: As stated above, virtually every drug overdose may be treated. In the case of Botox, an antidote is available should an overdose or misinjection be given to a patient. The antidote prevents additional muscle weakness but will not influence muscle weakness that has already occurred.

Dr. Mauriello's commentary: Dr. Mauriello has never had to treat a patient with an overdose of Botox®. He finds it safest to use the drug discretely and incrementally over several visits to determine the optimum dose. In this way, overdose is avoided. When the patient returns for retreatment several months later, the cumulative dose is injected in one treatment session.

As stated above, when large doses are given in the neck region, a single patient experienced problems with swallowing known as dysphagia. For this reason, low doses are given in the neck area not to exceed 30 to 40 units *(Carruthers J, Carruthers A: Practical cosmetic BOTOX techniques. J Cutaneous Med Surg 3:55-59, 1999 (suppl 4)).*

If some Botox is good, is more better?: The simple answer is "no." For any cosmetic procedure, it is far better to achieve a "good" response than to strive for a "superb" result and have a complication. The tolerance for problems with cosmetic surgery is very low.

> *Dr. Mauriello's commentary: A patient came into Dr. Mauriello's office and stated that she wanted to get the greatest effect from Botox. She requested additional injections after she was already treated in the incremental fashion outlined above. Increasing the dose of Botox once the optimum dose for any given patient is established is against Dr. Mauriello's philosophy. Adding more Botox will only increase the risks of additional side-effects. Certainly, increasing the Botox will not increase its duration of 3 to 6 months. If two aspirins relieve a headache, ten aspirins may cause side-effects.*

Dr. Mauriello's Treatment Philosophy: Dr. Mauriello attempts to determine the optimum dose for a specific area of the face in any given patient over two and sometimes three treatment sessions. Initial treatment requires injection of specific muscle groups to determine the effects of the Botox® on the particular individual receiving treatment. Photographic documentation allow Dr. Mauriello to analyze the effects of each treatment. Once that optimal dose is determined, reinjections at the same dose level are given in a single future office visit with predictable results. Dr. Mauriello encourages patients to wait 4 months between cosmetic injections. Repeat injections at short intervals are not advisable over time, and, although rarely, may lead to tolerance to the drug that hinder its effectiveness.

How effective is Botox® Cosmetic in Reducing wrinkles?
Allergen performed studies to determine the efficacy of Botox in treated the glabellar frown lines between the eyebrows above the nose.

The following data are provided by Allergan Pharmaceuticals (2525 Dupont Dr. Irvine, California 92612 through a subsidiary, Allergan Pharmaceuticals, Ireland Ltd.). In the Allergan-funded studies, frown lines were judged as "none," "mild," "moderate," or "severe." The ratings were performed 30 days after treatment. The response to the Botox was judged on a scale of "+4 to -4," where "+4" was considered complete improvement, and "-4," was considered "very marked worsening." For example, a moderate improvement was "+2 "(about 50%).

The participants in the study ranged in age from 22 to 78 years with a mean age of 46 years. Women represented 81.9% female of the study and 83.8% were white. Facial wrinkles were reduced up to 120 days.

The results of the Allergan sponsored study are summarized below:

Investigator's assessment	Severity of lines judged as "mild or none"
Day 7 after Botox	73.8%
Day 30	80.2%
Day 60	70.2%
Day 90	47.6%
Day 120	25.3%

Patient's or Subject's assessment	
Day 7	82.5%
Day 30	89.4%
Day 60	81.9%

| Day 90 | 63% |
| Day 120 | 39% |

As the Allergan data show, the patients experienced a subjective sense of a better response to the wrinkle treatment than did the investigators' assessment. During the 12-month study, 537 patients were evaluated. Four hundred and five patients obtained Botox ® injections, and 132 received a placebo. The study was double-blind in that neither the patients nor the investigating physicians were aware of which patients received Botox and which received the placebo (placebo group did not receive any Botox). During the first 8 months of the study, the maximum response rate occurred at day 30 after treatment. The investigators found that 80.2% of the subjects treated with BOTOX® COSMETIC, versus 3.0% of those subjects treated with placebo, responded to treatment. The criterion for response was reduction in the severity of glabellar lines at maximum frown. In addition, a significant improvement in brow furrow appearance (rated by the subject's self-assessment) also occurred in 89.4% of those treated with BOTOX® COSMETIC, and only 6.8% of the placebo group.

More marked improvement of 84.6% was experienced by patients less than 50 years of age. Marked improvement was 70.4% in patients aged 50 to 65, and 39.1% in patients over 65 years of age.

How long does it take for Botox to have an effect?
It generally takes 7 to 10 days. Patients may experience some relief almost immediately. In the majority of patients, the drug takes effect in 10 to 14 days. Each patient has a biologic response unique to his or her system. The results tend to be consistent for any given patient. In other words, if the drug starts working in 4 days, it will generally have an effect in 4 days on subsequent treatments.

How long does Botox work?

For any given patient, it usually lasts 3 to 6 months. If a patient has a result that lasts 6 months, that patient will generally experience the same result on subsequent treatments. Again, Dr. Mauriello recommends a return for re-treatment after at least 4 months.

How does Botox help patients with involuntary eyelid spasms?

Dr. Mauriello's interest is Botox is summarized by a list of publications and presentations below:

During Dr. Mauriello's fellowship in Oculoplastic Surgery at Will's Eye Hospital in 1982, patients with blepharospasm were often prescribed dark glasses and oral medications both of which provided little relief. The patients with severe blepharospasm were offered frontalis suspension (surgical suspension of the eyelids to the eyebrows) to help break the eyelid spasms. All patients with hemifacial spasm were considered possible candidates for neurosurgery, since oral pharmacologic agents rarely controlled the problem. Hemifacial spasm consists of involuntary muscular contractions that occur on one side of the face. It most commonly results from a tortuous vessel at the brainstem level that impinges on the seventh nerve that supplies one side of the face.

> *Dr. Mauriello visited Alan Scott, MD (Pacific Medical Center, San Francisco, California) who demonstrated the effectiveness of botulinum toxin in the treatment of blepharospasm and hemifacial spasm. Dr. Mauriello was one of the first physicians to bring this treatment to the New York metropolitan area in 1983.*

Dr. Mauriello was honored to be one of the original investigators of the National Institute of Health's study entitled Botulinum Toxin in the Treatment of Benign Essential Blepharospasm. This multicenter national center study was conducted from 1983–1989 and was headed by Dr. Scott. Dr. Mauriello was selected to act as a consultant to the Committee of Ophthalmic Procedures Assessment of the American Academy of Ophthalmology from 1985–89 to evaluate the effectiveness of botulinum toxin, type A, when the toxin was in its experimental stage.

Dr. Mauriello was invited to the Speaker's Bureau of Allergan Pharmaceutical (Irvine, California) in 1997. Since early 2000, he has been honored to serve as a Reviewer of the American Academy of Neurology's Therapeutics Assessment Subcommittee on Botulinum toxin therapy. He served on the Board of Medical Advisors of the Northern New Jersey Chapter of the national Benign Essential Blepharospasm Research Foundation from 1985–88.

What muscles will the doctor weaken to remove facial lines?
Wrinkles or rhytides are exaggerated by forceful contracture of muscles. Skin changes including loss of elasticity and ground substance in the dermis also cause wrinkles.

The muscle activity causing wrinkles is evident in the photographs below. *Botox works by selective temporary weakening of specific muscles that create wrinkles in a plane perpendicular to the action of the given muscle.* Knowledge of the anatomy is critical to the physician's successful use of Botox. Minimal doses of Botox® are optimally used in order to avoid weakening other nearby muscles that are not the target muscles that need to be treated to reduce the wrinkles.

The orbicularis oculi muscle is a superficial, circular muscle that encompasses the upper and lower lid and surrounds the eye. It closes the eyelid and pulls the brow down. The depressor supracilii is one of the muscles in the nasal group of muscles that along with the orbicularis oculi muscle, helps bring the nasal part of the brow downward.

The space between the eyebrows is widened after Botox. In order to decrease the forehead lines, the frontalis muscle, a brow elevator is weakened. Weakening the frontalis muscle may cause eyebrow drooping. Therefore, injections in anatomic sites adjacent to the frontalis muscle must be given discretely in order to avoid weakening of the eyebrow.

Treatment of vertical and oblique frown lines with Botox®
Wrinkles are improved by Botox. The effects generally last 3 to 6 months.

> *Dr. Mauriello has found over time in many patients that the effects are cumulative and do not result in loss of facial expression.*

Elevation of the eyebrow with Botox

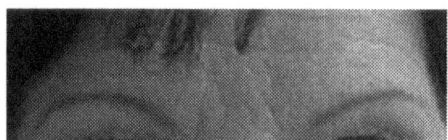   

Figure 3   **Figure 4**
BEFORE BOTOX   **AFTER BOTOX**

Before treatment (above left), the wrinkles above the brow and forehead are evident.
Widening of space between the eyebrows and the softening of vertical lines between eyebrows (above right) is apparent after treatment. The eyebrows also appear elevated in their outer aspect after treatment.

(Parts of photographs are obscured to maintain patient's confidentiality).

Should I have an eyebrow lift?

Many surgeons presently favor procedures that surgically elevate the eyebrows. Such procedures may be performed with small incisions in the scalp and facilitated by the use of endoscopes. However, it should be kept in mind that the eyebrow basically frames the entire face as well as the eyelids. Any change in contour and elevation of the eyebrows may change one's facial appearance. Eyebrow lifts, in Dr. Mauriello's opinion, are important when the brows are not at the same level.

Treatment of crow's feet (squint) lines with Botox®

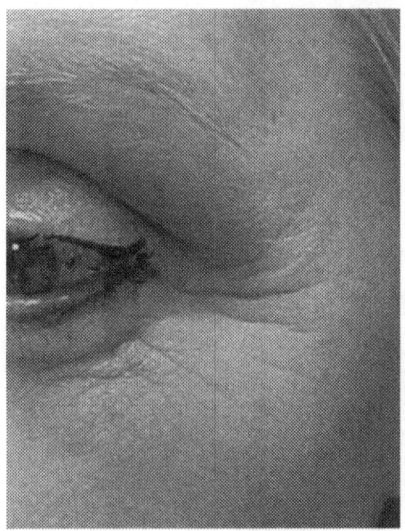
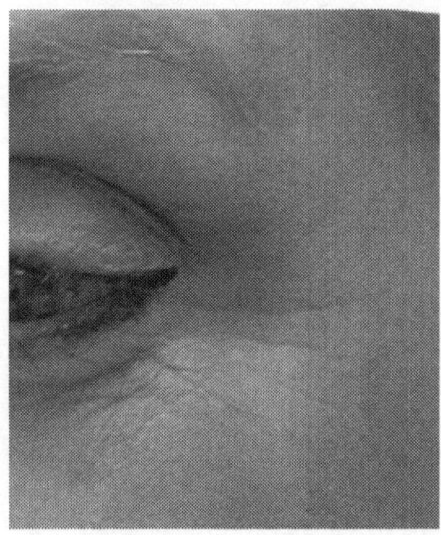

Figure 5
BEFORE BOTOX

Figure 6
AFTER BOTOX

Crow's feet (winkles lines in the corners on the eyes) may also be treated with Botox (above left). Subtle improvement may be seen in crow's feet after Botox treatment (above right). Patient is not smiling. Lower facial lines were not treated to avoid loss of facial expression.

> *Treatment of crow's feet may enhance the effects of upper ble-pharoplasty. Dynamic lines such as smile lines in the corner of the eyes (crow's feet) are optimally diminished by Botox®.*

There is still evidence of facial animation yet the lines in the corner of the eyes are diminished. Lower facial lines were not treated and the patient is, therefore, still able to smile.

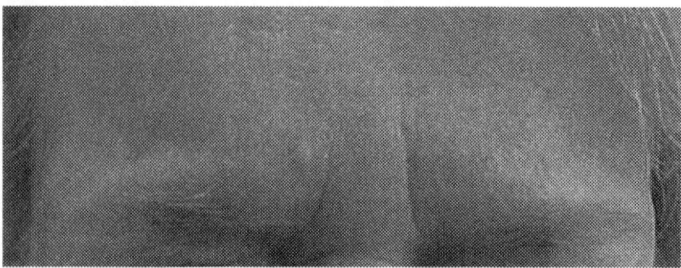

Figure 7
Vertical lines between eyebrows prior to first treatment with Botox.

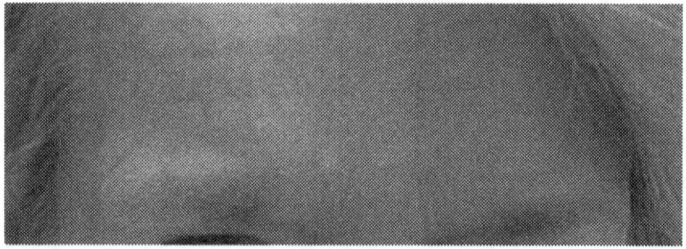

Figure 8
Just prior to fourth treatment, vertical lines between eyebrows are much less evident.

How is the treatment performed?
Your doctor will analyze your concerns and your particular facial musculature, and then treat those areas that may be improved. Photographic documentation of the eyelids and facial muscle, both with and without animation, are critical before and after treatment.

The procedure is performed in the office. After cleansing the skin, minute amounts of the reconstituted Botox ® are injected with a very small gauge needle. Generally, no anesthetic is necessary. Sometimes patients opt for ice application before and after the injections. The discomfort does not continue after the Botox ® is injected.

Dr. Mauriello's technique is to use the lowest dose to accomplish the purpose and thereby minimize complications. He sees patients at two-week intervals initially when they are first treated in order to determine the effect of minimal doses on specific muscle groups.

Once the appropriate muscle groups that are to be treated are determined along with the optimum dose, the injections are repeated at one treatment session. Injections are deferred for at least 4 months. There appears to be a cumulative effect of injections.

How do I help eliminate the nasolabial lines, marionette lines, and lipstick lines?
USE OF RESYTLANE®
While Botox® treatment is not ideal for the often deep lines that extend from the outer corners of the nostrils to the outer corners of the mouth (nasolabial folds), these lines are best treated presently with fillers such as collagen or hyaluronic acid such as Restylane (Medicis Aesthetics, Inc. Scottsdale, AZ 85258) FDA-approved.

Hyaluronic acid—the new dynamic filler is replacing collagen
A new treatment involves a drug known as Restylane. This drug was approved by the FDA in December, 2003.

Restylane is a synthetic compound, hyaluronic acid, that is a naturally occurring chemical known as a glycosaminoglycan (GAG). GAG is a vital component of all connective tissues. Hyaluronic acid may be thought of as the glue that holds the collagen in place. GAG's have water-binding capacities that enhance the effect of this filler material and correct wrinkles and skin foldings. GAG's decrease with age and benefit from replenishment. Presently this material is injected into the joints of patients with osteoporosis. Hyauronic acid is the material the fills the back of the eye, the vitreous.

Hyaluronic acid injections serve to replenish the loss of this matrix materially that occurs with aging. Hyaluronic acid is naturally occurring in rooster combs, bacterial cultures, umbilical cord, vitreous of the eye, tendons, and skin.

Unlike collagen, Restylane® requires no skin testing: Since hyaluronic acid has a uniform chemical structure throughout nature, there are no potential for immunologic reactions to Restylane. Collagen or bovine origin, in contrast, requires skin testing in the doctor's office to determine whether an individual is sensitive. The patient must wait 4 weeks after testing to determine whether there is a reaction. This testing is not necessary with Restylane. Hyaluronic acid is degraded very quickly within 1 to 2 days by the body's enzyme and then is converted to carbon dioxide and water in the liver.

Restylane is produced in various concentrations that have specific uses to reduce wrinkles:

Restylane Fine Lines—at 20 mg/ml concentration, contains 200 gel particles per ml is

> Treat fine superficial lines (For superficial dermis)

Restylane—100-gel particles per milliliter

> Treat deeper wrinkles such as eyebrow folds, deep lines that extend from the outer corners of the nostrils to the outer corners of the mouth (nasolabial lines) and is also used as a lip filler (For the mid-dermis)

Perlane—8-gel particles per ml

> For the junction of lower dermis and subcutis
>
> Treat deep folds in the nasolabial area and as a lip filler

Perlane Plus—4-gel particles per ml (most viscous or thickest form)

Restylane lasts for 6 months or longer as compared to collagen that last 3 to 6 months. The material is administered with a fine 30-gauge needle into the wrinkles in the skin.

Suggested Reading
Skin care

Bridenstine JB and Carniol PJ. Managing Postresurfacing complications
Laser skin rejuvenation Carniol PJ (ed) Lippincott-Raven, Philadephia, PA, pp243-260, 1998

Glaser DA. Patient preparation for resurfacing. Laser skin rejuvenation Carniol PJ (ed) Lippincott-Raven, Philadephia, PA, pp.87-102, 1998

Weinstein C. Combined carbon dioxide laser resurfacing with other facial rejuvenation procedures. Laser skin rejuvenation Carniol PJ (ed) Lippincott-Raven, Philadephia, PA, pp215-232, 1998

Mauriello JA. Editorial commentary on Incisional laser blepharoplasty and laser skin resurfacing, Khan JA in <u>Unfavorable Results of Eyelid and Lacrimal Surgery Prevention and Management,</u> Chapter 2, 53-54. Mauriello JA (ed); Butterworth-Heinemann, Boston, Mass, 2000.

Guenther LC. Optimizing treatment with topical tazarotene. *Am J Clin Dermatol.* 4:197-202, 2003.

BOTOX® and Restylane®
Mauriello JA. Blepharospasm, Meige syndrome, and hemi-facial spasm: treatment with botulinum toxin. *Neurology* 35: 1949–1500, 1985.

Mauriello, JA, Coniaris, Haupt E. Use of botulinum toxin in the treatment of one hundred patients with facial dyskinesias. *Ophthalmology* 94:976-79, 1987.

Mauriello JA, Aljian JA. Natural history of the treatment of facial dyskinesias with botulinum toxin: A study of 50 consecutive patients over 7 years. *British Journal Ophthalmology* 75:737-739, 1991.

Mauriello JA et al. Treatment profile of 239 patients with blepharospasm and Meige syndrome over 11 years. *British Journal Ophthalmology* 80:1073-75, 1996.

Mauriello JA et al. Treatment choices of 119 patients with hemifacial spasm over 11 years. *Clinical Neurology and Neurosurgery* 98:213-6, 1996.

Mauriello et al. Drug associated dyskinesias—a study of 238 patients. *Neuro-ophthalmology* 18:153-7, 1998.

Mauriello et al. Long-term enhancement of botulinum toxin injections by upper eyelid surgery in 14 patients with facial dyskinesias. *Archives Otolaryngology-Head and Neck Surgery* 125: 627-31, 1999.

Mauriello JA. Treatment of benign essential blepharospasm and hemifacial spasm: a preliminary study of 68 patients. In: *Advances in Ophthalmic Plastic Surgery* (Volume 4), Smith B and Bosniak S (eds); Pergammon Press, NY, NY, 1985, pp 283-289.
Mauriello et al. Oculinum therapy: its use in neuro-ophthalmology (Treatment of Facial Dyskinesia) in *Neuro-ophthalmological disorders,* Tusa R, Newman SA (ed); Marcel Dekker, 1994, 451-77.

Mauriello JA. Editorial commentary: Causes and treatment of blepharospasm: botulinum toxin, limited myectomy, and pharmacologic therapy on Surgical management of essential blepharospasm, Patel BCK, Anderson Rl. Chapter 8, 197-204 in *Unfavorable Results of Eyelid and Lacrimal Surgery Prevention and Management* Mauriello JA (ed); Butterworth Heinemann, Boston, MA, 2000.

Mauriello JA. Role of Botulinum Toxin Type A (**BTX-A**) (**Botox®**) in the Management of Blepharospasm and Hemifacial Spasm. *Scientific and Therapeutic Aspects of Botulinum Toxin*, ed. Brin M, Lippincott, Williams, & Wilkins, Philadelphia, Pa 2001.

Mauriello, JA. Techniques of Cosmetic Eyelid Surgery: A case study approach. Lippincott Williams & Wilkins, Philadelphia, Pa. 2004.

Section 6

PATIENT TESTIMONIALS: THE PATIENT'S PERSPECTIVE

CHAPTER 8

What can I learn from other patients who have undergone surgery?

While the insights of a surgeon are valuable, the experience is truly that of the patient. This chapter focuses on the patient's experience and their perception of the entire surgical experience.

PATIENT QUESTIONNAIRE: (only answer those questions which you are capable of, skip ones that you are not sure of)

PRIOR TO SURGERY:

1. Did you have any misconceptions going into surgery? Please comment.

2. What information would you like prior to surgery that you did not receive?

DURING THE ACTUAL SURGICAL EXPERIENCE AT THE HOSPITAL\SAME DAY SURGERY UNIT

1. What was the most surprising part of the surgery?

2. How much pain did you remember where "10" is the worse back-ache or toothache, "6" is the pain of small cut, and "0" is no pain?

3. What was the worst part of the surgical experience?

4. How did you feel after surgery in the recovery room and at home the first day?

EXPERIENCE AFTER SURGERY

1. Were you prepared for the degree of swelling and post-operative care?
   Please comment.

2. After surgery, did you have a change in outlook, attitude, and appearance?

3. Were there other changes in your life after surgery?

4. What was the greater benefit to your appearance?
   The upper lid surgery_____
   The lower eyelid surgery_____
   why?

5. What was the worst part of the post-operative experience?

6. How do you feel after surgery?
   Younger_____
   Refreshed_____
   Older _____
   No change_____

7. How many days after surgery, did you resume:
   wearing makeup   (if applicable) _____days
   work   (if applicable) _____days
   normal full activity   _____days
   vigorous exercise (if applicable) _____days

8. Please comment on any tips you might suggest for patients to make their experience less traumatic. Kindly please provide any comments about the following days after surgery:
   Day 1 after surgery_____
   Day 3 after surgery_____
   Day 7 after surgery_____
   Day 10 after surgery_____
   Day 14 after surgery_____

9. How long did it take for the scars to be imperceptible?

10. Did any scars not completely resolve?

11. How long did the tightness last?

12. What aspect of the final result could be better?

13. What was greatest functional benefit?
    Reading
    Driving
    Watching television

14. Would you have surgery again?

COSMETIC EYELID SURGERY—THE PATIENT PERSPECTIVE—A STUDY OF 27 PATIENTS

Dr. Mauriello presented the perspective of 27 patients (24 woman and 3 men) at the 2001 meeting of the American Society of Ophthalmic Plastic and Reconstructive Surgery. These results have been helpful to Dr. Mauriello and new patients seeking information about cosmetic eyelids surgery. The results were subsequently published as well (Mauriello JA: Cosmetic eyelid surgery—The patient perspective—A retrospective review of 27 Patients: <u>Ophthalm Plast Reconstruc Surg</u> 19:320-322, 2003).

All 27 pts were satisfied with the results and no surgical revisions were performed in this series. Twenty-six of 27 pts would opt for surgery again. A single patient who underwent 4-lid blepharoplasty was pleased with the final result, but did not wish to experience the unusual severe, post-operative eyelid edema that lasted several weeks.

Fifteen patients felt "refreshed" while 8 pts also felt "younger." No patient complained about a change in the shape of the eyelids. No patient complained that their eyelids were rejuvenated to a greater degree than the unoperated remainder of their face

Concerns of patients during preoperative consultation
During the pre-operative consultation, all patients wished to maintain or restore the shape of their eyes prior to surgery. Almost all patients asked about scarring, post-operative care necessary after surgery, and when normal activities could be resumed after surgery.

Intra-operative experience
All 27 patients felt prepared for the events that occurred on the day of surgery.

Post-operative course
AMOUNT OF POST-OPERATIVE DISCOMFORT
Little pain was experienced throughout the post-operative period.
On a scale of 1–10 where 10 was the most severe pain, "6" was the pain of cut, and "0" was no pain, the median pain experienced after surgery was 4.7).

Three patients specifically requested more details about the 1st week after surgery. Post-operative swelling and discomfort were more than expected in 4 pts. The assistance of someone the first night of surgery was strongly recommended by many patients. Two patients complained that their eyes

were covered in recovery room when ice applied A single patient was "surprised" that the bruising of the eyelid skin lasted several days.

Final post-operative scarring was not a concern of any of the 27 patients. *Tightness in the eyelid tissues especially the lateral canthus (outer corner of the eye) lasted 7 and 8 months, in 2 patients.*

Patients specifically commented that the effect of the cosmetic eyelid surgery was "to open their eyes"
Two patients expressed particular satisfaction that their surgeon was one who specialized in eyelid surgery

Patients returned to work a mean of 13.5 days (median of 7 days) after surgery
Eye make-up was applied a mean of 26 days (median of 21 days) after surgery.
Full activity was resumed a mean 21.9 days (median of 14 days) after surgery

Conclusions of study

Cosmetic blepharoplasty is perceived by patients as a means of facial rejuvenation that specifically restores their eyelids so that they appear refreshed

Patients experience minimal scarring and pain after cosmetic eyelid surgery

Complications were not significant and no secondary surgery was necessary in this series of 27 consecutive pts

Patients note that the effect of cosmetic eyelid surgery is to open the eyes rather than to change the shape of the eyelids

Preoperative patient education is instrumental in assuring pt accept-ance particularly about unanticipated eyelid swelling and bruising

The latter conclusion is one of the main reasons this book was writ-ten.

Comments are generously provided by patients who have undergone cosmetic eyelid surgery. Excerpts in the patient's own words are taken from their responses to a pointed questionnaire. The comments from patients are organized according to the specific type of surgery as out-lined below:

I. Combined upper lid blepharoplasty and repair of ptosis or eyelid droop
(Functional upper lid blepharoplasty and functional ptosis repair by levator advancement)

II. Combined upper lid ptosis and upper lid blepharoplasty and cosmetic lower lid bepharoplasty

III. Combined functional upper eyelid blepharoplasty and cosmetic lower lid blepharoplasty

IV. Lower eyelid blepharoplasty (**removal of bags and excess skin of the lower eyelids**)

V. Combined Cosmetic upper and lower eyelid blepharoplasty

The patient's personal comments are arranged by category:

I. COMBINED UPPER LID BLEPHAROPLASTY AND REPAIR OF PTOSIS OR EYELID DROOP (Removal of excess skin and fat in the upper lid and elevation of the eyelid margin above the pupil)
Comment by Dr. Mauriello

In individuals with a true blepharoptosis, surgical elevation of the eyelid margin (bleparoptosis repair) above the pupil is sufficient to improve vision. At the same time, excess skin which overrides the eyelid margin is excised (upper eyelid blepharoplasty). The excess skin is exaggerated as the eyelid margin is elevated.

Patients do not always opt for elective and cosmetic lower eyelid blepharoplasty since they may be only interested in functional improvement in vision or they do not wish to incur the cost of the cosmetic lower eyelid blepharoplasty. (Please refer to *Section 2: PREOPERATIVE EXPERIENCE, Chapter 3: Choice of Eyelid and Upper Facial Surgery and Alternative Treatments).*

The comments of the patients are grouped according to their age as follows (some comments are edited):

1. less than 40 years of age
2. 40 to 50 years of age
3. 50 to 65 years of age
4. 65 years of age or older

I. Combined upper lid blepharoplasty and repair of ptosis or eyelid droop
(Functional upper lid blepharoplasty and functional ptosis repair by levator advancement)

Editor's note: This group of patients is necessarily old.

Man—65 years of age or older
Dear Dr. Mauriello
I had eye surgery on my upper lids. The surgery was performed on both sides. My vision has improved 100%. I feel mentally great, physically great.

Thank you Dr. Mauriello

Man—65 years of age or older
Dear Dr. Mauriello:
My driving was difficult prior to ptosis (elevation of the eyelid margin above the pupil) surgery. Within a few days after surgery, I was able to drive at night without a problem. Oncoming lights do not look like sun bursts. On the golf course, I can now follow the ball while before my playing partners had to watch my ball (in order for me to find it after a shot). While watching television, I do not have to raise my eyelids to see as I did before surgery.

Woman—65 years of age or older
Dear Dr. Mauriello:
Immediately after surgery, the pain was a 6 out of 10 (where 6 is the pain of a small cut). I experienced discomfort that continued longer than I expected but overall I was told what to expect and had no major misconceptions.

In the recovery room and the first day, I did not like not being able to see because of nonstop use of cold compresses over both eyes.

The worst part of the entire surgery was the facial discoloration and stiffness of the eyelids that lasted longer than a month. I resumed normal full activity after 15 days.

After surgery, I had a better appearance, improvement in vision, and I no longer feel the need to raise my eyebrows in order to see more clearly. Reading, driving, and watching television improved 7 to 10 days after surgery. I look younger and do not look tired.

II. Combined functional upper eyelid blepharoptosis repair and blepharoplasty and cosmetic lower lid blepharoplasty
    Editor's note: Again, this group of patients is necessarily old.

Woman—50 to 65 years of age
Dear Dr. Mauriello:
MY REASONS FOR PLASTIC SURGERY
I decided to have plastic surgery on my eyes because of heaviness of the eyelids and difficulty reading.

INITIAL CONSULTATION
The information that I was given was very detailed. I did not have any misconceptions going into surgery.

POSTOPERATIVE COURSE
Everything around the face was uncomfortable because of swelling and bruising especially the first day. It is helpful to have some one to help you. The worst part of the postoperative experience was waiting for the swelling and bruising to disappear. The ice and Tylenol by mouth are helpful in relieving the temporary discomfort.

The most surprising part of the surgery was the first time I looked at myself in the mirror after surgery

I resumed normal full activity after 7 days. The tightness lasted 3 weeks. The greatest functional benefit has been my ability to read. I also feel refreshed. There was no scars and no aspect of the final result could be better. I would have surgery again if needed.

> **Comment by Dr. Mauriello:** *This particular patient had a brief episode of bleeding after surgery and was observed in the recovery room. Surprisingly, she did not mention this experience.*

Woman—65 years of age or older
Dear Dr. Mauriello:
MY REASONS FOR PLASTIC SURGERY
I decided to have plastic surgery on my eyes because of heaviness of the eyelids and difficulty reading.

INITIAL CONSULTATION
Dr. Mauriello explained the procedure thoroughly.

POSTOPERATIVE COURSE
I was most aware of swelling and discoloration of the eyelids the first day. The most surprising part of the surgery was the pressure on the face. On a scale of 0 to 10, where 10 was the worst backache, I had a 3. I was able to go home the day of surgery without discomfort. I felt good after the first visit to Dr. Mauriello.

AFTER SURGERY
The puffiness of the lower eyelids was gone and my eyes appear larger. I look younger and refreshed and would have the surgery again.

Woman—65 years of age or older
Dear Dr. Mauriello:
I had no misconceptions going into surgery.

I had pain during the surgery and was uncomfortable in the recovery room.

After surgery, I did not look tired and looked better. I resumed normal full activity 14 days after surgery and waited to wear makeup for 21 days.

It took about 4 weeks for the scars to be imperceptible and for the tightness (of the eyelids) to dissipate.

I enjoyed reading, driving and watching television. I look younger. I was less sore by day 7 and better by day 10 and felt well at day 14. I would have the surgery again.

Man—50 to 65 years of age
Dear Dr. Mauriello:
I had somewhat tired, swollen eyes the first day.

After surgery and everything healed, I enjoy watching television, driving and reading with improved peripheral vision and the eyelid skin no longer hangs over the eyes. My eyes look open and awake and I look refreshed.

I am no longer tired after reading by the end of a full working day. The results were excellent.

Woman—50 to 65 years of age
Dear Dr. Mauriello:
The most surprising part of the actual surgery was that I thought the surgery would take longer than it actually did. I had no misconceptions. The worst part was that my lids felt heavy after surgery. I felt tired in the

recovery room and at home the first day. The day after surgery, it is a good idea to rest and use the ice packs

I knew there would be swelling and I would be black and blue. I assumed that the ice would cure the swelling and it did. I resumed normal full activity for 5 days but no vigorous exercise

Ten days after surgery, I was in a club fashion show.

The tightness lasted 14 days. I was then able to read, drive, and watch TV.

II. COMBINED UPPER LID PTOSIS AND UPPER LID BLEPHARO-PLASTY AND COSMETIC LOWER LID BLEPHAROPLASTY
Man—65 years of age or older
Dear Dr. Mauriello:
I had upper lid surgery because of lines obstructed my vision. Before surgery, these lines disappeared when I lifted my eyelids with my fingers.

I had no misconceptions going into surgery but would have benefited from a better description of the whole surgical process ahead of time. There was minimal discomfort but the worst part of the surgical experience was the anticipation the day of surgery. I feel refreshed and younger and am extremely pleased with the lower eyelid surgery because of the drastic results. I no longer see any lines in my field of vision.

I resumed full activity in one to 2 weeks. I would undergo surgery if needed from the point of view of upper eyelid affecting vision.

Comment by Dr. Mauriello: *The importance of being prepared for surgery is highlighted in the above patient's comments is a common thread in almost all responses.*

Woman—50 to 65 years of age
Dear Dr. Mauriello:

The surgery that was performed on my upper eyelids was necessary. The skin on my upper lids became so loose and heavy that my eyelids were drooping and interfering with my vision. Since the surgery, my field of vision improved. I am now able to read again without pain or encumbrance. This improvement is very important to me because I am an English teacher and read extensively.

Woman—65 years of age or older
Dear Dr. Mauriello:

The eyelid surgery took longer than expected since I had previous cataract surgery which seemed shorter. I was very tired after surgery and took naps every day for 3 weeks. The eyeball was tender and especially sore when I washed my face but overall the pain was not very bad. I was not fully prepared for the degree of redness of the eyelids that lasted several days.

After surgery, it is important to have a system for using the hot compresses. As Dr. Mauriello suggested, I sat by the sink to apply heat after the eyelids were healed.

Now that the healing is over, I feel greatly refreshed. The scars were not noticeable after 2 weeks. I can now read better and would definitely have surgery again. I had dryness of the lower eyelids but that was not very uncomfortable. I was able to return to full activity after 14 days.

Comment by Dr. Mauriello: *The first week, it may be better to apply cooled boiled water rather than hot water from the tap to* *avoid wound contamination until the eyelid sutures are dissolved or are removed.*

Woman—65 years of age or older
Dear Dr. Mauriello:
I had absolutely no pain after surgery and no misconceptions prior to the surgery. Before surgery, my right upper eyelid was lower than my left upper lid.

Overall, after surgery, I am able to see better in the distance after my eyelids were elevated. I feel refreshed.

The tightness lasted 2 to 3 months. I experienced some dryness of the eyes after surgery that was partially relieved by eye drops (topical over the counter-lubricants).

Woman—65 years of age or older
Dear Dr. Mauriello:
I assumed I'd be working, driving, and looking normal within 3 weeks. I wish I had been told that some people do not heal quickly and that I would be such a patient. I had swelling that was extreme and lasted for a few months. I wore makeup in 30 to 45 days, returned to work in 10–14 days and resumed normal full activity and vigorous exercise in 2 to 3 months

I have no scars but still have tightness after 8 months.

> **Comment by Dr. Mauriello:** *This patient had an excellent result. However, in any given patient, the rate healing is unpredictable in terms of the amount of swelling and bruising and the amount and duration of healing which accounts for the*

tightness after surgery. To explain this uncertainty is a major reason why this book was written.

Man—65 years of age or older

Dear Dr. Mauriello:

I was very pleased with the operation on my eyes. After surgery, I have a greater area of vision and I also experienced about 50% reduction in tearing in both eyes. Both these factors make the surgery worthwhile. Before the surgery, the margins of my upper eyelids were covered by skin. When I look in the mirror now, I can see my upper lids.

I was never aware of any scars. I had tightness for 3 weeks or so.

I experienced no pain after surgery. I had double vision for about one hour after the surgery and I felt pretty normal. I was prepared for even more swelling. I appear less tired looking around my eyes and appear younger and refreshed. I started to play tennis 14 days after surgery and resumed normal full activity two days after surgery.

I would have the surgery again, if needed. Dr. Mauriello, thank you for your help.

> **Comment by Dr. Mauriello:** *Tearing may result from multiple causes. At times excess skin overhanging the upper eyelid margins interferes with the blink and, therefore, the tear film. Tearing results. It is important to distinguish patients with true ptosis in which simply elevating the eyelid margin by advancement the levator aponeurosis (blepharoptosis repair) from excess upper lid skin (dermatochalasis). In patients with excess skin, the blepharoplasty may improve tearing. In almost any patient who undergoes ptosis repair, excess skin will result due to an accordion effect in which the skin bunches up as the eyelid*

is elevated. Insurance companies only consider skin that over-hangs the lashes as functional even through a blepharoplasty should almost always accompany a ptosis repair. In such patients, the blepharoplasty component is considered cosmetic.

Woman—50 to 65 years of age
Dear Dr. Mauriello:
I would have liked more information on the aftermath of surgery. There was an aching and soreness for 4 to 5 days. The night of the surgery, I slept half sitting up. Bending over caused pressured, some bleeding, and headache for 14 days after surgery. The day after surgery I started getting up slowly. The tightness lasted about 7 months. The scars started fading about 30 to 45 days after surgery.

The greatest functional benefit is driving and watching television. The eyelids feel light and I feel refreshed. Frequent calls from Dr. Mauriello's office and the staff at operating room site were helpful.

IV. LOWER EYELID BLEPHAROPLASTY (removal of bags and excess skin of the lower eyelids)
Woman—50 to 65 years of age
Young woman
Dear Dr. Mauriello:
I had no misconceptions going into surgery. I had general anesthesia due to combined nasal surgery and was nauseous from the general anesthesia. The results were visible in 2 to 3 days. A pulling sensation occurred when moving my eyes for the first week after surgery. The ice in the glove the first four days after surgery did not put excessive pressure on the eyelid skin.

Since the surgery I feel refreshed and have a better mental attitude. I would definitely have lower eyelid surgery again.

Woman—less than 45 years of age

Dear Dr. Mauriello:

I had baggy lower lids that really affected my appearance.

The surgery you performed removed the bags. I now look younger, refreshed, and (have) a better attitude towards life.

V. COMBINED COSMETIC UPPER AND LOWER EYELID BLEPHAROPLASTY

Comment by Dr. Mauriello

Studies have shown that cosmetic surgery benefits more than just appearance. The positive change in quality in life is highly significant. In a paper presented at the 12th Annual Congress of the International Confederation for Plastic, Reconstructive, and Aesthetic surgery, 105 cosmetic surgery patients between the ages of 18 and 70 were included. Their level of their depression, quality of life, coping skills, and personal resources were assessed at periodic intervals: 2 weeks before surgery, 2 months, and finally 6 months after surgery. A highly significant change was evident in all variables 6 months after surgery.

Woman—less than 45 years of age

Dear Dr. Mauriello:

MY REASONS FOR PLASTIC SURGERY

I decided to have plastic surgery on my eyes for several reasons. I was not interested in changing my appearance drastically and only wanted a fresher, perhaps younger look.

I have very prominent bags under my eyes and I also have very heavy brows. I had no upper eyelid area at all above my eyelashes. I constantly look tired and older than my 45 years.

OTHER ALTERNATIVES TO SURGERY
After trying every cream and lotion that promised to reduce the puffi-ness and dark circles under my eye to no avail, I decided to look into plastic surgery.

SEARCHING FOR A SURGEON
I researched and checked the credentials of several plastic surgeons. After several consultations, I made my final decision to have my surgery performed by Dr. Mauriello based on recommendations from family members and friends who were former patients of Dr. Mauriello. One friend had the same kind of plastic surgery was interested in and the other had reconstructive performed because of skin cancer in the eye area. I also based my decision on Dr. Mauriello's professionalism and willingness to answer my questions and concerns. I had confidence in him and, most importantly, felt comfortable with him.

PRESURGICAL CONSULTATION
At my consultation with Dr. Mauriello, we discussed what procedure would be used for my surgery and the type of anesthesia.

I made my decision to proceed with the surgery several days later after the consultation based on pictures that I was shown of other patients who had similar operations. It was decided that I would have all 4 lids done. I initially was only concerned with my lower lids, but during the consultation, and looking at other patients, I realized that having only the upper lids done would not be sufficient. It made much more sense to have all lids done to achieve the desired results.

I was told I would need at least one week recovery for the worst of the swelling and to go down, but that it would take months for my eyes to return to normal.

DATE OF SURGERY—Operative experience
The operation was performed in the fall at 9:00 under local anesthesia. There was a certain amount of minimal pain that I had not anticipated, but overall the procedure was without complications and other rather quickly. The only thing I was unprepared for at the time was double vision after the operation. Dr. Mauriello told me that was probably due to local anesthesia and to make sure that I did not leave the hospital until the double vision had cleared up, which it did in approximately 45 minutes.

Overall, the surgery was successful and uncomplicated. I was given all the information I needed to make an informed decision about the procedure. The staff at the (free standing surgical facility was informative and extremely helpful. The entire experience was, in general, what I was told it would be.

POSTOPERATIVE COURSE
in the recovery room the day of surgery, I was tired and a little uncomfortable that continued into the next day. Although I was not in pain, I was not prepared for the discomfort that was short-lived. I was given adequate medication for the discomfort that I did have. The swelling made it difficult to see for several days. From days 3 to 7 after surgery, the eyes did not close and tears drops were used to keep the eyes moist since they were a little sore and dry.

Within a week after surgery my appearance was vastly improved. The swelling was all but gone but the eyelids felt a little tight (photograph). Some the discomfort was noted but short lived.

It took a full two weeks before the most severe of the discoloration disappeared and the swelling was almost unnoticeable. By Day 14 after surgery, there were no real signs that I had surgery. Some slight swelling and tightness were still noticeable. My eyes continued to running at times (but the tearing was improved by topical tears). The stitches were a little uncomfortable.

I was able to wear makeup in 21 days, return to work in 7 days and resume normal full activity in 14 days and vigorous exercise in 21 days.

It has now been 4 months since the operation, I could not be more pleased. The circles and bags under my eyes are gone and my upper lids look better than they ever have. I feel more confident. The main improvement is that the puffiness of the eyelids is gone. I was not looking for a drastic change in my appearance. I achieved the result that I was hoping for. I no longer look tired all the time and I believe that I look "refreshed," if not exactly younger.

I would have the surgery, but I won't need it. I still have slight scarring around the edges of my eyes, but I have been told that in time these too will fade.

To anyone contemplating this procedure, I would recommend researching carefully, finding a doctor you are comfortable with and trust, and have realistic expectations.

Comment by Dr. Mauriello
This patient was quite happy with the result but she experienced dry eye symptoms that caused tearing. These symptoms were treated with topical over-the-counter tears until they subsided.

Woman—40 to 50 years of age
Dear Dr. Mauriello:
I would like a more detailed step-by-step procedure from the time entering the facility to when I left the recovery room at the freestanding surgery center. The pain was similar in degree to that of a small cut. The worst part of the surgery was in the recovery room and vagueness of what was going on around me. After care should be explained prior to surgery not in recovery room when too drowsy and confused.

The first day after surgery is uncomfortable at home and you really need someone at home to help you. I was not fully prepared for swelling. I had difficulty sleeping. I would have been more prepared had I read about other patient's experience. It is helpful to speak to others who had surgery.

Two months after surgery, I had no perceptible scars. The tightness of the eyelids lasted for about 3 to 4 weeks.

I am very happy with my result. It is very positive result, smooth and my eyes are more youthful (Photographs).

Comment by Dr. Mauriello
The request for a step by step analysis of the surgical experience prompted the writing of this book.

Woman—less than 45 years of age
Dear Dr. Mauriello:
The most painful part of the procedure was removal of fat in lower eyelids. I remember the bright lights at the end of the surgery and the deep ache in the lower eyelids the day of surgery.

I felt surprisingly well in the recovery room and at home the first day. I had great energy, sat with friends, talked, and ate a large a large dinner the day after with no desire for a nap. I did not feel at all bad.

I was prepared for the degree of swelling since I had a previous nasal surgery and knew what to expect.

After my eyelids completely healed, I had an uplift of spirit and well-being. Since I feel I look better, I feel better about myself. I look refreshed from the lower eyelid surgery and look less tired. The upper lid skin that was taken off was like taking age off.

I wore makeup 7 days after surgery and chose to return to worked in 21 days but resumed normal, full activity in 7 to 14 days and vigorous exercise after 28 days. I resumed contact lens wearing after 21 to 28 days and had a lot of dryness around my eyes until about 10 weeks after surgery.

The scars were fully imperceptible after 12 weeks. All scars completely resolved. I had tightness in the eyelid area for 10 weeks following surgery. There was also occasional blurry vision at night for several weeks. I would have the surgery again but the swelling of the lower eyelids took 10 to 12 weeks to disappear.

Comment by Dr. Mauriello
In general contacts lens cannot be worse for two to three weeks after surgery or until almost all eyelid swelling returns to normal.

Woman—40 to 50 years of age
Dear Dr. Mauriello
I had no misconceptions going into surgery and experienced no pain but a feeling of eyelid tightness after surgery.

During the surgery, I felt no pain but I heard taking.

I had a reaction to stitches which caused itching along my upper incision line. The day after surgery, one should expect swelling, redness, bruising, and appearing ugly. The results are excellent. I had less swelling 7 days after surgery and by day 10 after surgery, the redness and bruising subsided. By day 14, the appearance was much improved.

I feel refreshed and was able to wear make-up in 8 to 10 days, work in 5 days, and resume vigorous exercise in 12 to 14 days. I enjoyed an improved subtle change in my appearance and my eyes looked more open.

Comment by Dr. Mauriello
The comments below are those of a patient who had surgery elsewhere and was referred to me. She was extremely unhappy due to severe dry eye that were so severe she was unable to work or function at all comfortably. Her unhappy experience is rare but occurs when patients with dry eye do not feel fully prepared for discomfort and its appropriate treatment after surgery.
Younger woman
I have dry eye and sought another opinion after cosmetic eyelid surgery. I wished I had been warned about dry eye.

I had no pain at all after surgery but was nauseous as I was being driven home without sunglasses. I wanted to be in dark room and wished I had not traveled so far after surgery.

I had to use hourly drops (topical lubricating tears 0 after surgery for two weeks.

My result shows that my left lower eyelid is slightly pulled down. Dr. Mauriello recommended I wait 6 months to a year for any further surgery.

Comment by Dr. Mauriello
The need to delay revision of eyelid surgery is usually advisable unless the eyeball is exposed and at risk. With time, the healing usually helps improves any asymmetries. Additional surgery may only add to further eyelid scarring and delay return to normal daily activity.

Woman—less than 40 years of age
Dear Dr. Mauriello:

The worst part was not being able to see well due to bandages and ice immediately after surgery.

I have the following recommendations after surgery:

Day 1 rest don't bend
Day 3 take it slow
Day 7 resume almost full activity
Day 10 go out and enjoy your new appearance

I would have surgery again. It took 2 years for all the scars to be imperceptible.
The tightness lasted a few days.

I feel refreshed and look younger and the basic shape of my eyelids has not changed.

Younger woman

Dear Dr. Mauriello:

I had no misconceptions prior to surgery and I believe my expectations were realistic. I had complete confidence in you.

The most surprising part of the surgery was being totally out of it on the way home and the shock of how swollen my eyes looked the first few days. I would rate my discomfort as 4 out of 10 and it was not actually pain.

The worst part of the surgical experience was, perhaps, some anxiety the morning of surgery.

I have a total fog after surgery and on the way home. It was good to just go to sleep and wake up more alert. While carefully advised of postoperative care, I really was not fully expecting the degree of swelling and overall discomfort.

My outlook and attitude were always positive. The appearance around my eyelids improved after surgery and this was most important to me.

The removal of the excess skin of the upper lids made the eyes appear larger, brighter, and more open. The lower eyelid surgery resulted in a subtle "lift" and overall better look.

After surgery, I know feel more refreshed and positive about my eyes and appearance.

I wore make-up eye and face makeup 14 to 16 days after surgery. I went to work in 5 days which was a stretch but manageable. I resumed normal full activity in 7 to 10 days and vigorous activity in 10 days.

My suggestions after surgery:

Day 1 plan total rest, some extra assistance is recommended.

Day 3 plan to get out for short periods and have dark glasses that you enjoy wearing after surgery.

Day 7 resume a regular schedule with a slower pace.

Day 14 resume a full schedule and start to exercise.

It took several months for the scars to be almost imperceptible. The redness of the incisions may continue. The tightness in my eyelids lasted for months and after a year I still feel some tightness.

I have total satisfaction. I would have this surgery again but never a face lift. Ideally, you should be realistic. Essentially you will not change your appearance that much and the change and improvement is most evident to you, personally, not family and friends.

It is important to have supportive friends and family and to realize that surgery is an intense process and patience is required during recuperation.

Comment by Dr. Mauriello
Eyelid surgery restores symmetry to a small anatomic unit and, therefore, the results are longer lasting than after a face lift.

Woman—40 to 50 years of age
Dear Dr. Mauriello

My (upper) eyelids started to droop over my eye. It started to bother me some. Some days I woke up and they were swollen.

I had a hard time seeing to drive and had to push my lids up.

I went for a consultation with Dr. Mauriello. He tested my eyes and saw that the lid was blocking my vision.

My vision improved after surgery.

Comment by Dr. Mauriello
The following patient had surgery elsewhere and had severe dry eye and an uncomfortable post-operative course. She was treated by me after surgery. Had the treatment been instituted earlier, she probably would have been happier.

Woman—40 to 50 years of age
Dear Dr. Mauriello:
I had the great misconception that having my eyes done was nothing, "a piece of cake." The worst part of the procedure was that the pain in my eyes was like poison ivy with nails in my eyes. The swelling was not a problem. I was unable to wear make-up for six weeks.

I recommend that you investigate the doctor, his credentials, and his experience in performing eyelid surgery. I am happy with the final result but I never realized there were doctors who specialized only in eyes.

Woman—40 to 50 years of age
Dear Dr. Mauriello:
I had drooping upper eyelids and my peripheral vision was greatly improved after surgery and I look younger. I was able to wear makeup in 2 to 3 weeks and returned to work in 10 days (as a nurse) but normal full activity in 2 days.

There was no post-op pain or bruising or black and blue at all.
I look younger and refreshed and would have surgery if needed

Woman—40 to 50 years of age
Dear Dr. Mauriello
Thank you Dr. Mauriello for giving me my life back.

APPENDIX

Definition of Common Eyelid Terms (functional glossary)

atrophy—thinning of a tissue with its normal elements such as fat atrophy of face with aging

blepharon—(Greek) eyelid

blepharoplasty—surgery to repair a defect or correct the eyelid for improve both form and function of the eyelid—cosmetic eyelid surgery, cosmetic eyelid lift (also known as "cosmetic eyelid surgery")

collagen—fibrous tissue produced by fibroblast cells in the dermis.

canthus—corner of the eye
     medial (nasal) canthus—corner of the eye by the nose
     lateral (temporal) canthus—corner of the eye by the ear

canthopexy—surgical procedure which supports and elevates the inner or outer corners of the eye. A secondary effect is to tighten the skin of the lower eyelid.

commissure—the point where the upper and lower eyelids meet—
   medial (nasal) commissure by the nose
   lateral (temporal commissure) by the ear

conjunctiva—clear layer that extends over sclera and has a potential space, the subconjunctival space that may fill with blood or fluid due to inflammation as often occurs after surgery. The conjunctiva "joins" the eyelid to the eyeball.

   transconjunctival lower lid blepharoplasty—the incision is bag in through the conjunctiva in the space between the eyelid and eyelid

cornea—outer, front of the eye is an optically clear specialized fibrous tissue (or watch glass) that covers iris (colored part of iris) and is continuous with the white fibrous protective coat of sclera. Its epithelium is non-keratinized (does not contain keratin).

cosmetic eyelid surgery—see blepharoplasty

crow's feet—wrinkles in the outer corner of the eye. These wrinkles may be static, present when the individual does not smile and dynamic and present upon smiling

dermis—consists of the layers under the overlying superficial lining cells
   The more superficial dermis is the papillary dermis which supports the skin while the deeper dermis is the reticular dermis. Carbon dioxide laser resurfacing that destroys the reticular dermis

will cause permanent scarring while damage to the papillary dermis promotes new collagen that thickens the skin

edema—fluid that accumulates in tissues after surgery

epidermis—outer layer of cells that line the superficial skin

epithelium—outer layer of cells that line any structure
    The eye surface has conjunctival epithelium and corneal epithelium. These surfaces do not produce keratin since they are mucosal surfaces

erythema—redness is one of the three hallmarks of inflammation, heat, rubor (redness), swelling, and increased temperature due to an increased rate of cellular metabolism. May be due to thermal injury as after carbon dioxide laser or to inflammation induced by the trauma of eyelid surgery

exposure keratitis—exposure of the cornea and drying of the cornea which if untreated may lead to corneal erosion, ulceration, and infection

eyebrow and forehead musculature
    glabella—area between eyebrows
    corrugator muscle—muscle just above brow that creates frown lines

    procerus muscle—muscle that brings brow down and arises from radix (base of nose and inserts into forehead

    frontalis muscle—muscle of entire forehead, elevates eyebrow, and creates horizontal furrows

eyelid

> lower eyelid—from the lower eyelid margin to the inferior orbital rim (bone under the eye)

> upper eyelid—from the upper eyelid margin to lower aspect of the eyebrow. It is responsible for 75–90% of eyelid closure.

eyelid skin—thinnest skin in the body and only placed where muscle is directly underlying the skin with no intervening fat. Elsewhere in the face, such as the cheek, there is fat between the dermis and underlying facial muscles.

fibrous tissue—scar (collagen) tissue produced by fibroblasts in order to heal wounds

folds—normal anatomic depressions that may become exaggeratedly deepened with age due to drooping of surrounding tissues and atrophy or thinning of subcutaneous facial fat with age

> nasolabial—fold from corner of nostril to outer corner of mouth
> nasojugal—fold between side of nose and cheek (jugal)
> upper eyelid fold—excess skin that overhangs eyelid crease

hair follicles—are associated with sebaceous glands that express their sebum or oily into the lumen of the hair follicle to serve as an inherent cool cream for the lubrication of the overlying skin.

> The great number of pilosebaceous units distinguish facial from skin outside the face.
> The nose and forehead have more sebaceous units than the cheeks or temples.

lagophthalmos—inability to close the eyelids which may lead to exposure keratitis (exposure of the cornea and drying of the cornea which if untreated may lead to corneal erosion, ulceration, and infection)

levator aponeurosis—tendon of the levator muscle which creates the upper eyelid crease

levator muscle—muscle just below the orbital roof (bone above the eye) in the upper eyelid that elevates the upper eyelid.

limbus (corneo-scleral limbus)—circular junction of white sclera and clear cornea where conjunctiva ends and appears to surround iris

malar cheek (fat) pad—highest point of cheek or cheek prominence below the eye is composed of thickened fat under skin. This fat pad is elevated by Dr. Mauriello's small incision techniques during routine lower cosmetic blepharoplasty.

melanocyte—pigment cells in the skin responsible for melanin pigment production and the relative lightness (hypopigmented) or darkness (hyperpigmented) of one's skin

> Melanin in the epidermis of the skin, like melanin throughout the body, is produced by specialized a cell termed the melanocytes
> The melanin protects the skin surface against ultraviolet light by absorbing it
> For this reason, skin cancers do not occur in blacks and rarely in individuals
> With dark skin

midface—from inferior orbital rim (bone) to mouth

mongoloid slant—a mongoloid slant is such that the outer or lateral canthus of 2 mm of 2/25 of an inch above the medial canthus. With age, the lateral canthus descends and assumes an anti-mongoloid slant such that the outer corner of the eye is at the same level of below the level of the medial corner of the eye (medial canthus). Lower lid blepharoplasty should restore the mongoloid slant. Scarring after lower lid blepharoplasty may exacerbate the anti-mongoloid slant.

orbit—bone that houses the eyeball and consists of four walls each of which has a corresponding rim or projection of bone that can be felt on the surface of the face below the skin

> medial wall—on the side of the nose (medial orbital rim is not defined since the lacrimal drainage system or sac is located there)

> lateral wall—on the side of the ear (lateral orbital rim is a projection which projects the eye from its side)

> roof or superior wall—above eye (superior orbital rim is covered by the eyebrow)

> floor or inferior wall—below eye (inferior orbital rim is below eye)—fat bags prolapse above the inferior orbital rim

pigmentation in the skin—may be due to melanin which causes a tan or collection of blood and its breakdown products after surgery. Blepharoplasty does not remove skin pigmentation or melanin or dark circles in the skin under the eye

plastic surgery—surgery that is characterized by repair of a defect and restoration of apart that affects the form and function of that part.

ptosis-droop
>   blepharoptosis—droop of the upper eyelid margin
>   brow ptosis—droop of eyebrow
>   lash ptosis—downward pointing of the eyelashes over the pupil

reticular dermis—deeper and thicker reticular (net-like structure) layer which when penetrated by the laser during laser resurfacing may result in permanent scarring of the skin

sclera—outermost fibrous protective coat of the eye whose front extension is the clear cornea

scleral show—usually an undesirable result after cosmetic blepharoplasty in which white sclera is seen under the limbus of the eye or colored iris

stratum corneum—The outermost layer of skin or epidermis is composed of epithelial cells which have a protective role. This horny layer which is produced by the epidermis is composed of keratin. The keratin in the stratum corneum protects against physical damage but also to some extent against sun exposure and is most developed on the palms of the hands and the soles of the feet. The eye surface, like all mucosal surfaces in the body, is not keratinized (does not contain keratin or the "horny" outer layer of skin).

tear trough deformity—space under the lower eyelid over the bone of the orbital rim due to gravitational downward sagging of the cheek. The deformity creates shadows under the eyes

0-595-16846-9

www.ingramcontent.com/pod-product-compliance
Lightning Source LLC
Chambersburg PA
CBHW061348280526
45784CB00001B/183